Published by Gina Nelson Media LLC

264 El Rancho Road

Kalispell, Montana, 59901

www.ginanelsonmedia.com

ISBN: 9798224045792

First Edition

MEDICAL ASSISTANT DELUXE

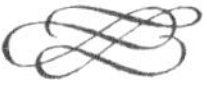

GINA NELSON, M.D.

GINA NELSON MEDIA LLC

ACKNOWLEDGMENTS

I would like to thank my teachers, professors, attending physicians, fellow physicians, nurse colleagues, and medical assistants.

Most of all, I would like to thank my patients.

CONTENTS

PREFACE

I'm Dr. Gina Nelson. I have been an obstetrician gynecologist since 1994. As I write, I am a dying breed. I am a private practice OBGYN. Being in private practice means that I am self employed, as opposed to being the employee of a hospital or a hospital system.

Once upon a time, almost all physicians were in private practice. According to the August 16, 2022 edition of the Journal of the American Medical Association, JAMA, in 2012, only 5.6% of physicians were hospital employees. Fast forward to 2022 and an estimated 74 percent of practicing physicians have become employees of either a hospital or a corporate health system. This is part of what is called hospital consolidation.

In this short decade, the institutional dynamics in medicine have changed enormously. Before, private physicians would answer to their professional colleges, the courts, market forces, and their patients. Now, more often than not, they answer to corporate administrators. The lines of account-ability have been completely re-drawn.

I have come full circle and back again. In 1994, I finished residency and landed in a small northern town with a respectable community hospital. There was no practice for me to join, so I had to hang out my own shingle. Residency had not prepared me for this. Fortunately, I had a savvy and supportive father-in-law who shepherded me through not only my early practice but my early practice management as well. I lucked out with my first batch of staff, and we launched a successful private practice for the first female OBGYN in the area, me.

My residency was grueling. Private practice, by contrast, seemed easy. Patients were eager to support the first women in the area and the practice filled. We felt like we were on some sort of vanguard. My staff enjoyed high autonomy and employed their skills with creativity. Patients were loyal. Nowadays, our practice would have been considered a "boutique" style of practice, with personalized, responsive, and continuous care over long periods of time.

As the years passed, the pressures of being on call all the time for our private patients wore me down. The recession of 2008 taxed our resources. Back then, there was no Affordable Care Act (ACA), and while money came in, it did so in fits and starts. We kept seeing our long-term patients, even if they could scarcely pay.

By 2010, my friend and mentor, the CEO of the hospital, suggested I lay aside the burden of private practice and become a hospital physician. She persisted, and in 2015, the appeal of call coverage and a consistent paycheck resulted in the practice's purchase and me joining the hospital. It did not work out as planned.

For one, my CEO friend sickened and passed away from breast cancer. For two, the call coverage never materialized. For three, the paycheck came with a heavy dose of uninformed input into the workings of a practice in obstetrics and gynecology, which hospital administration had never managed. For example, they never adjusted to how we sometimes needed to drop everything and run to labor and delivery, relying on office staff to deal with the patients left behind.

There was other unwelcome meddling. For instance, administration had a tendency to move staff around like chess pieces. People are not chess pieces. Relationships could scarcely be formed. Learning could not be consolidated. This tactic alone sullied the spirit of the office. It seemed like administration had never heard of the adage, "if it ain't broke, don't fix it."

These same external forces acted on my sister offices. Administration's stated goal was to create "one big happy family" of obstetrics and gynecology, a cohesive service line, but it backfired. The department splintered, and in 2020, I returned to private practice. Fortunately, our patients stayed with us through both transitions.

Many things changed between 2015 and 2020. These all affected the reestablishment of my private practice. In 2020, the real estate market was buyer friendly and interest rates had fallen. In that climate, I purchased an ideal office space across the street from our old one. It was a bit of good fortune.

The renovation this space needed gave me the chance to indulge myself. We wanted an office space that would be comforting, beautiful and eclectic. I did not hold back. Crystal chandeliers and silvered deer skulls went up without hesitation. Aromatherapy and high end speakers were standard for each room, a great departure from hospital austerity.

Software changed in the same time interval. Payroll, once a substantial burden, became a breeze and our electronic medical record (EMR) became more streamlined. Social media had matured, and all the staff were digital natives. We ditched the clunky software of the hospital in favor of the streamlined Apple Macintosh (Mac) based software of the open market.

Pressure on hospital staff related to consolidation caused many medical assistants to leave or be let go. This worked in my favor. These medical assistants were eager to continue working, but in private environments, if possible. These environments conferred more of a sense of job security, and staff enjoyed more creative autonomy. With the new larger office space, we needed more staff, and plenty were available.

While employed, I lost touch with my staff. When private again, the camaraderie returned. Everyone felt much more secure.

With the camaraderie came good performance, even though many of the new staff needed teaching. Some were certified nursing assistants (CNAs) transitioning to medical assistants (MAs). Some were from different disciplines and some were just freshly minted. Teaching once again became enshrined in the practice, as it had been before.

This time around, I have put some of those teachings in writing. This volume is for my MAs and those that work with them. Indeed, this work provides a guide for women's health paraprofessionals of any kind, whether they be MAs, CNAs, Licensed Practical Nurses (LPNs), registered nurses (RNs), Nurse Practitioners (NP), or Physician Assistants (PAs).

DISCLAIMER

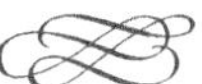

People in medical training, from phlebotomists to physicians, will quickly come to understand that *medicine is an art as well as a science*. It is complex, imperfect, and moving forward as quickly as possible. Very little is "cookbook". This means that very little is simple or formulaic. It may seem so at first glance, but it is not.

To approach a patient in order to take a history, perform a physical, or obtain specimens, is to recognize that your work will end up as part of a body of information used eventually to make a diagnosis and prescribe a treatment. Rarely does one piece of this puzzle tell the whole story. But each piece is important.

Understanding this leads to an understanding of disclaimers. Disclaimers are a means for writers and health care providers to avoid unfair medico-legal liability. However, they are also a tool for understanding. The disclaimer reminds readers and users that a written document cannot tell the whole story. It is to remind readers that a book lacks the clinical context of a specific patient. A book is to teach general principles and practices; it is not meant nor can it ever be, comprehensive in scope. Therefore, the author and publisher of this guide assume no responsibility for any inaccuracies, errors, or omissions, or for any consequences arising from the use of the information in this guide.

THIS INFORMATION IS DESIGNED as an educational resource to aid clinicians in their training as they learn about providing women's health care, and the use of this information is voluntary. It should not be considered as inclusive of all proper treatments or methods of care or as a statement of the standard of care. It is not intended to substitute for the independent professional judgment of the treating clinician. Variations in practice may be warranted when, in the reasonable judgment of the treating clinician, such course of action is indicated by the condition of the patient, limitations of available resources, or advances in knowledge or technology.

THE INFORMATION PROVIDED in this guide is intended for educational purposes only and is not a substitute for professional medical advice, instruction, diagnosis, or treatment. This guide does not establish a doctor-patient relationship and is not intended to be used for medical emergencies. Always take the advice of a licensed medical professional for any questions or concerns you may have regarding your health, or the health of others. Do not disregard or delay seeking medical advice based on the information contained in this guide.

· · ·

WHILE THE AUTHOR of this book makes every effort to present accurate and reliable information, this publication is provided "as is" without any warranty of accuracy, reliability, or otherwise, either express or implied. Gina Nelson Media LLC and Gina Nelson MD PC do not guarantee, warrant, or endorse the products or services of any firm, organization, or person.

WE WILL NOT BE liable for any loss, damage, or claim with respect to any liabilities, including direct, special, indirect, or consequential damages, incurred in connection with this publication or reliance on the information presented.

WHO IS THE MA?

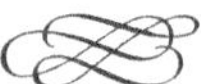

I am the doctor, the obstetrician gynecologist. But who is the medical assistant? Who is she to herself and who is she to the patient?

TRAINING for medical assistants varies widely. Some who have been working for a while become quite specialized. Roles range from taking vitals and rooming patients to substantial teaching capacity.

THE MA SHOULD THINK of herself as a protector. She protects both the doctors and the patients. Between the doctor, the front office, and the medical assistant, the patient should get all that she needs from her appointment.

SOMETIMES, doctors are rushed, absent, or unapproachable. The MA mitigates these things. However, the MA does not have all the answers. She cannot do exams or procedures. This is where the doctor becomes her resource. The MA and the doctor are a dyad, a pair, a duo. They must work together in a coordinated fashion to optimize both their professional lives and the care of the patients.

IN THE PATIENT'S VIEW, the medical assistant is the right hand of the doctor. Patients often confuse the types of medical assistants which offices use. These can range from CNAs or nurses (LPNs or RNs) or actual MAs. It is important for medical assistants to clarify their title and position to patients. More importantly, it is important to understand that patients sometimes credit them with an enormous amount of knowledge which they may or may not possess. This volume, while directed at medical assistants, may be of benefit to anyone in healthcare who takes care of women. Any forthcoming references to medical assistant may be understood as applying to anyone performing these roles.

THE MA BRIDGES TWO WORLDS, **the medical and the administrative.** While the doctor must know the pathophysiology of Group B strep (GBS) disease, the medical assistant must know the correct swab to test for it and where to find it in the office. Moreover, she must be familiar with any constraints associated with the submission of the specimen. She must label it, transport it, and order it in the computer, all without error.

THE MEDICAL ASSISTANT also bridges the two realms of the back office and the front office. She ensures that the doctor's orders are executed correctly. She assists the front with referrals, procedures, prescriptions and orders.

IN SHORT, the medical assistant is the glue that binds the office together. She helps bind patients to the doctor, and the medical with the clerical. Her importance should not be underestimated.

TECHNICAL RESPONSIBILITIES
OF THE MA

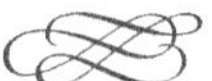

The tasks of receiving patients, rooming patients and recording vital signs are deceptively simple. They hide the crafting of a relationship between MA and patient. Through this relationship, patients are educated, issues are unearthed, and problems are addressed.

ALL THE WHILE, as she moves through the office doing these "simple" tasks, the MA gets an overview of the front office and the back office, and how they are functioning together. You will not find a more valuable observer.

RECEIVING AND ROOMING PATIENTS

Greeting the patients seems simple. It is as simple as going to a party and meeting each of the diverse guests in attendance. Some people will be gregarious and others aloof. Some will be know-it-alls and some will be terrified. The MA has to be the perfect host. She has to say something to put each unique guest at ease.

. . .

ONCE SHE GREETS THE PATIENT, the MA sees to her physical comfort. Does she have a heavy coat? Is she struggling with small children? It is often courteous and useful to offer the patients water at this stage. A urinalysis (UA) will be needed, and the water can help hydrate and relax the patient. The MA guides the patient in from the waiting room. From there she can take her purse, diaper bag, and finally her shoes. She places these in her exam room. The patient, unencumbered and literally unweighted, can be weighed and her chief complaint and vitals taken.

RECORDING THE CHIEF COMPLAINT (CC)

The chief complaint is a brief statement, often a single phrase or sentence, which informs the doctor of the basic reason the patient is there. It is something that the MA must write in the chart and convey to the doctor. It would be easy if it were the first words out of the patient's mouth. Often it is not. Sometimes it takes a few minutes of open-ended conversation to deduce the gist of the reason for the visit.

ONCE IN A WHILE, the patient does not want to discuss the chief complaint with the MA. The MA should not take this personally. She just needs to let the doctor know in advance that she will need to take time to review the chart before the visit, so that, in the absence of a chief complaint, she does not go in completely uninformed. The MA needs to get enough information into the chief complaint to orient the doctor, but not take so much time that it detracts from the visit or gets the clinic behind.

VITAL SIGNS

The measurement of vital signs is real medicine. Vital signs comprise height, weight, blood pressure, pulse, respirations, and temperature. These vital signs tell a great deal about the patient. Every medical assistant should attain expert status in these things. Every office should have highly reliable equipment for these measurements.

WHILE EACH MEDICAL assistant should develop her own preferences for the order in which these things are done, there are some precedents to consider. There are many tricks an MA can use to foster efficiency and accuracy. For example, many offices now have a tiny finger mounted pulse oximeter which also reads out the pulse. This can be placed on the finger at the very beginning of the measurement of the vital signs. While this is sitting on the index finger, blood pressure can be taken. All the while, a thermometer can be in the patient's mouth.

PULSE

Devices like the pulse ox are useful, but have a tradeoff. Taking the pulse manually may give you more information. For example, a manual taking of the pulse allows you to feel several other features. Is the pulse weak, thready, or strong? Importantly, taking a manual pulse offers you the critical information about whether the pulse is regular. You may detect atrial fibrillation, bigeminy, or trigeminy just by putting your index finger on someone's pulse.

.   .   .

It won't take long for any medical assistant to get a feel for the range of pulses in different people. They will soon learn that fit individuals have a lower resting pulse. We speak of a resting pulse as though it is the pulse that we get when a patient is sitting on one of our exam tables. Technically, a resting pulse is the one that we obtain when we first awaken from sleep before we stir.

MAs will also notice that pregnant patients have higher pulses. The careful observer will also notice that there is more pulse pressure. We call this a hyperdynamic state, and it is normal, to a degree, in pregnancy.

This hyperdynamic state is common in certain illnesses, too. Sometimes a patient will say, "I thought my heart was going to beat right out of my chest." Those types of comments are clinically relevant and can make informative additions to the medical record.

Medical assistants will note that the definition of bradycardia is a consistent pulse under 60, while the definition of tachycardia is a pulse greater than 100. If that seems like a pretty wide range, it is. It reflects the great expanse between those who are quite fit, and those that are severely de-conditioned.

The pulse reflects more than the level of conditioning at hand. It can reflect an acute disease process, most notably infection. An increase in pulse due to infection may be due to fever. Any time the core temperature goes up, the pulse rises too. This is called the Q10 effect. The rate of chemical reactions in the body increases with increasing body temperature. This affects the whole body including the circulatory system and the heart, which produces the pulse.

METABOLISM IS REALLY JUST **the collection of chemical and enzymatic reactions in the human body.** Therefore, it is no surprise that our metabolism increases with increasing temperature. Our heartbeat is a primary indicator of our metabolism. If we have a temperature, our heart rate will, all other things being equal, increase.

INCREASED pulse can reflect low volume. In our bodies, this usually means dehydration. In the world of obstetrics and gynecology, it can also mean anemia or blood loss. The body knows it has to get a certain amount of oxygen to the tissues. If this delivery of oxygen is compromised due to lack of fluid volume in the circulatory tree, the system will compensate by increasing the pulse to deliver what little fluid volume there is more rapidly. If there is a scarcity of oxygen carrying red blood cells in an otherwise normal blood volume, the system will again compensate to deliver the right amount of oxygen to the tissues by increasing the pulse. A scarcity of red blood cells in the blood is called anemia.

ONE CAN HAVE DIMINISHED oxygen carrying capacity in other ways besides anemia. Sometimes there are plenty of red blood cells, but their carrying capacity is diminished due to lack of iron. Just about everyone remembers basic high school science, wherein we learned that the oxygen-carrying molecule in the red blood cell is hemoglobin. To make effective hemoglobin, one must have adequate iron. Those who are iron deficient may have plenty of red blood cells, but those cells are going to be pale and marginally effective at carrying oxygen for lack of adequate hemoglobin, which is red.

PULSE OX

Pulse oxygenation, or pulse ox for short, is coming into focus as a relevant vital sign. Unfortunately, this relates to two relatively recent phenomena: the increasingly prevalent diagnosis of obstructive sleep apnea (OSA) in women, and the upper respiratory infection associated with COVID infection. During sleep apnea, people obstruct their own airway during sleep and their oxygen levels fall. This causes strain on the system over time. It can lead to higher blood pressure and increased risks of cardiovascular disease.

MANY TYPES of upper respiratory infections can lead to lower oxygen status. Normally, when this occurs, the patient feels miserable. However, COVID has posed different challenges, in that many people have showed low oxygen levels with minimal symptoms. This phenomenon has been dubbed "happy hypoxia".

BLOOD PRESSURE

Taking blood pressure is something that everyone should learn to do. Ordinarily, illness declares itself through symptoms. However, high blood pressure does not. Adults who are entirely symptom free may have elevated blood pressure and not know it. This is why high blood pressure should be checked routinely, even in the absence of symptoms. High blood pressure has been called the "silent killer" because it can cause damage to vital organs before causing symptoms.

In clinic, blood pressure should be taken at every visit. Some people say that patients should be settled before blood pressure is taken. Others have argued they shouldn't be. We are, after all, interested in what their blood pressure is under all circumstances. By this logic, we should poke them with pins before we take the blood pressure. My opinion is that coming to the doctor is provocation enough. Patients have to drive through traffic, wait in a waiting room, talk about their insurance or lack of it, and get poked and prodded.

BLOOD PRESSURE IS a rough description of the flow of blood in the vascular tree, from departure out of the heart down to the finest capillaries in the toes. The top number, the systolic blood pressure, is the peak pressure as the heart pumps one beat. As the heart rests between beats, the flow in the vessels ebbs. At the lowest, weakest flow, the pressure is at the diastolic pressure.

TO TAKE BLOOD PRESSURE, an occlusive band is fitted around the upper arm. The band has a pressure gauge. Done manually, a hand pump is used to inflate the band so it squeezes the arm. Simultaneously, the MA applies a stethoscope and listens for the flow within a large downstream vessel. When the stethoscope is on the vessel, and the band fully inflated, there is no sound, since the vessel is squeezed off and there is no flow from the pulse. Then, the pressure on the band is gradually relieved at a rate of about 3 mm Hg per second. When the first pulse sound appears, the MA notes the pressure on the gauge. This is when the pressure of the blood exceeds the pressure of the band. This is the systolic pressure. As the pressure on the band is progressively reduced, the blood will flow ever more freely. When the sound of the pulse disappears, the pressure on the gauge is noted. That is the diastolic pressure in the vessel, the lowest pressure that is in the vessel at that moment.

WE REPORT the blood pressure as systolic over diastolic. You can quickly get a feel for the range of pressures to which a patient's vessels are exposed. Ideally, systolic blood pressure should be less than 130 and diastolic blood pressure should be under 80. Chronically high values can damage vessels over time. Damaged vessels lead to a variety of disease processes, like heart attacks and stroke.

ONCE BLOOD PRESSURE IS TAKEN, it is recorded in the chart. It is also verbally reported to the patient. This is so that she will develop a sense of what her blood pressure values normally are. If they deviate from her normal, she will be the first to know.

OFTEN PEOPLE ARE incredulous at the blood pressure values that are obtained in clinic. They protest that their blood pressure is usually not that high. It is best to believe them and agree. This is an opportunity to explain that blood pressure varies with circumstances. Patients like this should be advised to obtain a home blood pressure cuff, aka sphygmomanometer, perhaps an automatic one. You can even get ones which are bluetooth connected to a smartphone for easy and accurate recording of measurements over time. In this way, they can convince themselves of the situation.

. . .

IF YOU KEEP GETTING values higher than others, check the fit of your cuff. Larger patients may require a larger cuff. *A cuff which is too small will give artificially high readings.* It is also worth calibrating your cuff against others.

ONCE IN A WHILE a patient will come in feeling "WADAO". This is a snarky but useful acronym for "weak and dizzy all over". This set of symptoms needs to be taken seriously and thoroughly investigated, most likely in an acute care setting such as the Emergency Room (ER). However, patients presenting this way to clinic can begin their workup with vital signs. In particular, they can be subjected to orthostatic vital signs. This is a set of vitals to see if a patient is adequately perfused.

BEING PERFUSED MEANS GETTING enough blood circulation to the body. If someone is poorly perfused, they may feel WADAO. If someone is unsure if they are WADAO, orthostatic vital signs will settle it. Orthostatic vital signs are basically BP and pulse taken three times, once laying down (supine), once sitting up, and once standing up, in that order. One takes these after the patient has been in each position for at least a couple of minutes. If the BP falls too much or the pulse increases too much after any of the position changes, the patient is said to be orthostatic. If there are symptoms of lightheadedness with the position changes, they are orthostatic. Certainly, if they faint, they are orthostatic. If they are orthostatic, they are said to "tilt", another useful slang term from the Emergency Room. Said one doctor to another, "Does she tilt?"

TEMPERATURE

In these days of COVID, temperature is of particular importance. It has always been important. Elevations in temperature most commonly accompany infection. This can be respiratory infection but also urinary tract infection, especially once it has gone into the kidneys. Typically, a simple bladder infection will not cause an elevation in temperature.

ALL VITAL SIGNS, but especially temperature, take on special importance when dealing with postpartum and post-op patients. One is always on the lookout for infections in postpartum patients. These particular patients are set-ups for infection. Their incisions, lacerations, blood loss and even their anesthesia puts them at risk for infections, usually at the uterus or surgical site, but also at old IV sites, the bladder, and in the lungs.

INFECTIONS DEEP IN THE BODY, for example, the pelvis, do not always show an elevated temp. In fact, one of the first vital signs to change during a deep infection is the pulse. Often, an elevated pulse will precede elevated temp as a harbinger of infection.

CORE TEMPERATURES ARE the most accurate. These are obtained from oral or rectal thermometers. Skin or even ear temps can reflect peripheral vasodilation or just being flushed and can give misleading values in either the high or low direction.

WEIGHT

The medical visit is a time of reconciliation with the facts. In that spirit, it is very important that we weigh all patients at every visit. "I am so looking forward to this" said precisely no one. People are concerned about their weight, but they have trouble confronting it. It is our job to help them confront it. We can do this by speaking to them in supportive terms, and by framing the issue as a manageable problem.

PATIENTS CANNOT ADEQUATELY MANAGE their weight unless they are aware of it. It has been more than adequately proven that quantifying an issue leads to the ability to control it. We here in the United States are in the middle of an obesity epidemic. We know that this plays into just about every other disease process imaginable, not just diabetes and heart disease, but orthopedic problems and cancer as well.

IT IS critical that the medical assistant be supportive of the patient no matter whether their weight is up, down, or the same as their last measurement. Try to have a "cup half full" attitude. Caregivers who find this part challenging should actually rehearse what they plan to say. It pays to go to a little extra effort to avoid hurting someone's feelings, alienating or paralyzing them. For example, if a heavy person's weight is down, the job is easy. They can be congratulated on their efforts.

IT BEARS REPEATING that it is the patient's efforts that should be praised rather than the absolute accomplishment itself.

· · ·

IF THE WEIGHT is unchanged and it is supposed to be down, one can always point out that at least it has not gone up. If the weight is up when it is supposed to be down, the caregiver should note the mood of the patient. If she is really frustrated with herself, the caregiver should counsel her not to be so hard on herself. If she is blasé, the caregiver might suggest food journaling, in order to discover what is sabotaging her efforts.

HEIGHT

The measurement of height seems unnecessary. However, it factors into BMI and is important for other reasons.

It should always be done in stocking feet. Before measuring height, check the patient's posture to make sure that it is normal. So many people have markedly bad posture that it is worth noticing. Take this opportunity to remind patients to stand up straight. It looks better, makes them feel more confident, and will prevent back issues and discomfort in the future.

OLDER PATIENTS MAY BE CONCERNED about a loss of height. This can be related to loss of bone density also known as osteoporosis or osteopenia. Osteoporosis can lead to vertebral compression fractures, which can lead to pain and disability. Patients who appear to have lost height should discuss it with the doctor.

BETWEEN HEIGHT AND WEIGHT, body mass index (BMI) can be calculated and recorded. While not a perfect index of anything, it is useful as a rough measurement of size.

VITAL SIGNS IN PREGNANCY

In pregnancy vital sign have particular significance. The maternal mortality crisis in the United States is due largely to hypertensive disorders of pregnancy.

HYPERTENSION IN PREGNANCY is often related to obesity, which may predate the pregnancy. We are therefore particularly careful to get accurate baseline vital signs in the first trimester of pregnancy and forward. With pre-pregnancy or early baseline weights and blood pressures in the chart, we can be quick to discern when subsequent values deviate into abnormal ranges.

IT IS interesting to note that in the second trimester, blood pressure (BP) naturally dips in all patients, even in those who are naturally hypertensive to begin with. In the third trimester, they naturally rise back up to their baseline values. It is also in the third trimester that they usually become abnormal if they are going to do so.

PREGNANCY AFFECTS PULSE. As previously noted, pregnant women are more "hyperdynamic" than non-pregnant women. This means the pulse is higher and more forceful. You can feel the increased dynamic nature of the heartbeat by simply placing your hand over the patient's heart. This is because, in pregnancy, the heart has to work harder to meet all the demands of the growing pregnancy and its infrastructure. These changes are reflections of the stereotypic adaptations of the cardiovascular system to pregnancy.

OFFICE MAINTENANCE

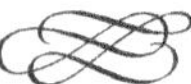

*T*he physical maintenance of the office is really everyone's responsibility. However, the medical assistants have a special obligation because the medical assistant's work is especially impacted by the layout and supply status of each room. The organization of the rooms either empowers or prevents the MA from doing their job.

THE MEDICAL ASSISTANTS clean and stock the rooms. They also sanitize and check it between each patient. They are the first to know if something is malfunctioning or if supplies are running low.

THOSE WHO STOCK the rooms should also organize the stored supplies. These same medical assistants are the ones who should keep inventory records to ensure that when supplies are low, they are replenished without interruption.

. . .

THE OFFICE MANAGER should assist the MA in keeping a central list of all the supplies that the office uses, where they are obtained, and at what cost. This will streamline shopping. If purchase dates are included, then the office can gauge how often they use certain things. Regular buying patterns can help with office budgeting.

SIGNAGE IN STORAGE areas can be helpful. Consistent storage spots with clear supply labels help everyone, especially new hires and fill in staff. Any instructions pertaining to the storage of certain supplies should be made into laminated cards and posted on the insides of cabinet doors. Expiration dates should be noted on all inventory items, both for best patient care and avoidance of waste. All of this falls under the purview of the clinical MAs with clerical help from the manager.

THE MAS ARE ALSO responsible for the office's disposal practices. Medical office waste is classified as white, red, and sharp. Red waste contains enough blood to drip or is infectious. Of course, all blood is considered infectious. Sharps are things like used needles, syringes, or scalpels. They go in special "sharps boxes" which are red. These are taken away by a dedicated disposal company that likely services many medical offices in your area. White waste is basically everything else - normal garbage. Housekeepers take care of white waste, while MAs take care of the red waste and the sharps.

LAUNDRY CAN BE HANDLED in many ways. If your office uses all disposables, then you have more garbage and no laundry. If your examination gowns and break room hand towels are cloth like ours, then laundry can be done either by a laundry service or by a member of the staff or housekeeping. This is provided they have access to a high temperature washing machine such as one would use for a commercial vacation rental. Soap, hot water, and perhaps a little bleach kills all that needs to be killed.

BEYOND THIS, everyone should be responsible for the orderliness of the office. Most offices have a housekeeping service to handle the heavy cleaning. In the housekeeper's absence, everyone pitches in to maintain the common areas. However, answering the phones and keeping the clinic running on time is paramount; office tidying is secondary.

INTRODUCTION TO DOCUMENTATION

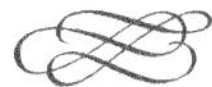

*M*edical record keeping is important for many reasons, from practice reimbursement to patient safety.

EVERYTHING THE MA DOES, from tasks like shots to phone calls, becomes part of the patient's medical and or legal record. Each one of these encounters, however brief, must be documented.

THE MEDICAL RECORD is central to the patient's care. It is the basis of billing. More importantly, it is the repository for your patient's health data. We have to think of our patient's aggregate and specific data as tools to use in fostering health and combatting disease. For example, a data point would be one set of blood pressure readings. By contrast, aggregate data would be a series of BP readings on the same patient over a decade. Aggregate data can be very revealing.

. . .

WE MUST ATTEND CAREFULLY to the data points which we include in the medical record. "Garbage in, garbage out" certainly applies here. *If we include high-quality data in the medical record, and a complete set of it, and we do this over time, we can see emerging trends on which we may intervene.* This is especially true with something like hypertension and diabetes, which are major killers in our country.

ALL MODERN HEALTH *care providers should think of themselves as data scientists.*

CLASSIC HISTORY TAKING

Physician directors or senior staff should train MAs in the classic note taking conventions. In obstetrics and gynecology, it is conventional to begin with a typical preamble of age, gravity, parity and either gestational age or last menstrual period. Gravida refers to the number of pregnancies of any kind that the patient has ever had, including failed pregnancies like miscarriages or ectopics. Parity, or para, is the number of deliveries that a patient has had, including anything after twenty weeks of gestation.

FROM THERE, a variety of classic history taking formats can store information. These range from a comprehensive history and physical used for a new patient annual visit to a procedure note tailored for a specific instance.

ONE OF THE most common formats is the SOAP note. SOAP stands for subjective, objective, assessment and plan. SOAP notes are used for episodic or problem oriented visits. They can also be used for postpartum or post operative documentation.

SOAP NOTES ARE NOT robust enough for an annual exam or a new OB appointment. Instead, a traditional history and physical (H and P) is necessary. While an MA will rarely find themselves in the position of charting an entire H and P on her own, it is helpful for her to understand how they are constructed.

THE HISTORY BEGINS with the chief complaint. This is a simple statement about why the patient is there. It is rarely more than one line. The MA records the chief complaint. From there, the full history is taken in a section called "history of present illness" or HPI for short. The HPI is taken by the principle caregiver.

THE HPI CAN DRAW in elements of the patient's history which directly pertain to the chief complaint. However, past medical history items are left for the past medical history section. Following HPI comes past medical history (PMH). It is broken down into past gyn history, past ob history, past medical (as in internal medicine) history, past surgical history, then medications and allergies. The history concludes with family history, social history and then the catch all, Review of Systems (ROS).

THE HPI really tells the patient's story. In HPI, we record how the patient has been in general. In our questioning, we proceed from the broad to the specific, asking more and more particular questions. For any given symptom, we want to ask about all the details, and all the modifiers. For example, we need to know when a symptom started, how long it lasted, what pattern it took, its intensity on a scale of 0 to 10, what made it better, and what made it worse, and so on.

WE INCLUDE pertinent positive and pertinent negatives. A pertinent positive is a symptom that the patient is having. A pertinent negative is a symptom that they do not have, which, by its absence, tells us something about their condition. For instance, if a patient reports a sore throat, that is a pertinent positive. If you ask her whether she had a fever, and she denies it, that is a pertinent negative.

GYNECOLOGY HISTORY (GYN HX)

After HPI, as an obstetrician gynecologist, I fill out the gyn section. Here, we discuss the facts and figures related to her menstruation. This includes her age at menarche, the first period, and the length of her interval.

MENSTRUAL INTERVAL IS the distance between the first day of one period and the first day of the next. Often, patients believe we are asking about the time between the end of one period to the beginning of the next. This is incorrect. The menstrual interval can tell us many things, so it is important to record it correctly.

THE GYN SECTION of history also includes information about the menstrual length and qualities such as its painfulness, crampiness, duration or volume. To understand menstrual volume, we remember that not everyone knows what everyone else's period is like. We usually try to quantify it using information about the physical methods that people use to handle their period, for example, tampons, pads, or menstrual cups.

THE GYN SECTION also includes information about any sexually transmitted infection (STI) history. This includes information about Pap smears and any resulting procedures like colposcopy. We should also note whether they have had the Gardasil vaccination to protect against human papillomavirus.

OBSTETRIC HISTORY (OB HX)

The ob section often takes the form of a grid, graph, or spreadsheet. This includes the delivery date, gestational age, birthweight, route of delivery, and any other pertinent issues.

MATTERS OF INTERPRETATION are left to the doctor, whereas facts and figures are best charted by the MA before the patient sees the doctor. Filling in the vitals, meds, allergies, delivery details and other such objective facts are perfect tasks for the MA to handle, so the doctor can get on with the things that only they can do.

PAST MEDICAL HISTORY (PMH)

Past medical history becomes a complex category to record, depending on the history. The physician should probably fill in the majority of the detail. That said, the medical assistant can record the general category of disease, for example, asthma. The caregiver can come in later and find out the age of onset, number of hospitalizations, intubations, and current asthma medication use.

PAST SURGICAL HISTORY (PSH)

Surgical history is often straightforward, including items like appendectomy and wisdom teeth extraction. However, certain types of surgical detail belong in the chart. For example, with appendectomy, or "appy" as it is often called, one must always note whether it was ruptured at the time of operation. This is because a ruptured appendix is likely to cause adhesions or scar tissue in the pelvis. This type of information is very important to any future surgeons who need to enter the abdomen or pelvis.

OTHER SURGICAL DETAILS which belong in the chart should include the side of a particular operation, such as right ovary versus left ovary. Any history of cancer surgery should include stage and grade of the tumor and a summary of its treatments. Many patients will not know this level of information off the top of their head. It may become necessary to glean this information from old records, such as operative (Op) notes.

ALLERGIES

Most EMRs have a well highlighted section on allergies. Notation of allergies usually falls to the MA. MAs should note that patients often confuse allergies with intolerances. Both should be listed in the EMR. Certain intolerances, while not allergies, can be serious.

.   .   .

PATIENTS FORGET their allergies more often than you might imagine. Modern EMRs have helped me notice that *people with allergies documented in the chart will often report that they have no allergies!*

CAREGIVERS SHOULD ASK before administering any drug whether a specific allergy to that drug is present. This should be done regardless of what the chart says. This is a good practice even with substances like Betadine or lidocaine, which MAs have occasion to administer.

REACTIONS TO ALLERGEN should be noted in the chart. These can range from mild to life threatening. A mild allergy is often heralded by a rash or itching of the lips. More serious allergies involve throat swelling and shortness of breath and even anaphylaxis and collapse. More detail on the reactions is better. MAs should note that mild allergies can worsen with age or repeated exposure to the antigen.

NAUSEA IS OFTEN REPORTED as an allergy, but technically, it is not one. An allergy is an immune reaction of a specific type and is potentially life threatening. Nausea is not an allergy. It is simply uncomfortable and unhelpful. Even so, clinicians want to know about such reactions and avoid them if possible, going so far as to include them in the allergy section of the chart.

SOCIAL HISTORY (SH)

Social history holds many keys to the patient. Traditionally, social history includes marital status, education, and employment history. It also includes substance use history for alcohol, drugs, and smoking. The American College of Obstetricians and Gynecologists (ACOG) also advises screening for abuse of all types. This data belongs in the social history.

DURING THIS PART of the history, caregivers may begin to understand the patient as a person. Social history, including level of educational attainment, allows us to grasp the patient's health literacy and capacity for self care.

HEALTH LITERACY IS **the amount of health related knowledge that the patient has.** Medical assistants, by self selection, have interest and education in aspects of human biology, disease, and the practice of medicine. They may not grasp the relatively low levels of health literacy in the general population. It is critical that they and the caregivers that they assist bridge this information gap.

FAMILY HISTORY (FH)

Family history becomes more and more meaningful as we recognize the genetic basis of disease. That said, we usually restrict our attention to first and second-degree relatives. A first-degree relative is a parent, sibling or child. A second-degree relative is a first-degree relative of a first-degree relative, for example, an aunt.

SOMETIMES WE CARE about relatives beyond first and second degree if they all have the same or related type of cancers. That is because there are some cancers with a genetic basis that fall in groups. We call these genetic groupings syndromes.

PATIENTS OFTEN CONFUSE CANCER TYPES. It is not uncommon for patients to call cervical dysplasia "cervical cancer". Ovary and uterus cancer are occasionally confused. This is understandable since women of older generations did not discuss the details of illness, especially if it involved reproductive organs. Prior to the 1960s, cancer was discussed in generic terms. The science of the day may not have permitted accurate identification of every tumor.

IT IS important to take Family History (FH) for non-cancer related conditions. Degenerative diseases like diabetes and hypertension may largely depend on lifestyle choices such as diet and smoking, but they are still more likely to take place in some families than others.

Even some obstetric conditions run in families. Mullerian abnormalities like uterine anomalies can run strongly in families. These abnormalities of the uterus can predispose to miscarriage and other problems like preterm labor. I have a couple of mother-daughter pairs in my practice who both have uterine anomalies and the complications associated with them.

IN SOME FAMILIES, women suffer from recurrent miscarriage. An anatomic uterine abnormality explains some of these cases. In others, it is a blood factor. Either way, a careful family history may reveal a treatable condition which can be caught before it can cause problems.

REVIEW OF SYSTEMS (ROS)

The doctor has to review all the history in every chart. The MA factors this in and fills in her part, according to the plan she has with her doctor. Review of systems is the fail-safe mechanism in this joint history taking scheme. It is an encyclopedic list of questions we ask the patient, either by asking her to fill out paperwork, or, more traditionally, by taking a verbal history.

ROS SKIMS over all the broad classes of symptoms in all the organ systems of the body. It is not uncommon for the review of systems to unearth something important that the patient failed to mention in her chief complaint.

WHEN I GET to this part of the history, I take a moment and explain to the patient that it is a general checklist that we must review to meet quality standards. Knowing this, one can review it quickly, and it does not seem so impersonal. Performing ROS is part of good history taking. It is also required in order to use certain higher-level reimbursement codes which the visit would deserve. The doctor, the MA, or both can review the ROS, depending on the arrangement.

COLLABORATION AND SCRIBING

MAs and doctors both contribute to the same chart, but they can do so in different ways. The MA and the doctor can work independently or concurrently on medical records. How they work together depends on their EMR, the electronic medical record, as well as many other variables.

. . .

IN THE INDEPENDENT SCENARIO, the MA reviews the patient's documents, takes a certain amount of history from her and loads it into the medical record before the physician sees the patient.

USING an MA as a scribe is an example of the MA and the physician working concurrently to acquire and input the medical history. Either can work well if tailored to the dynamics of the office.

MINIMALLY, in the independent scenario, the MA will input the reason for the visit, the chief complaint, and a set of vitals. She may also do pregnancy tests, urine dips, blood draws, and immunizations. In some settings, the MA then reviews any medical history forms which the patient has supplied. Using this, she can begin filling out the EMR. If she is sufficiently experienced, she may do her own history taking and fill in the EMR with more detail. The degree to which the history is taken can vary by the practice's needs. Once the MA has done all her preliminary work to whatever degree requested, the caregiver can take the patient, finalize the history, do the physical exam (PE) and make assessment and plans.

THE EXTENT to which the MA works alone or collaboratively is called out by the staffing and the clinic schedule. Ideally, regardless of the plan that is chosen, nothing is overly redundant. From this perspective, the MA and the doctor work as a pair.

. . .

ON THE OTHER HAND, the MA knows her history will be reviewed and completed by the caregiver. This type of redundancy is beneficial. Two heads are better than one.

SOMETIMES THE MA may be interrupted in her history taking since the doctor is ready for the patient. The physician may not want to wait for the MA to finish her part of the patient's history. This too, should be in the interests of clinic flow.

IF THIS METHOD is done poorly, both members of the team will feel inefficient. Done well, the duo can complement each other's efforts. Each team pair need to find their sweet spot. They may have to realize that their collaborative sweet spot can vary from patient to patient.

IN THE SCRIBING SYSTEM, the physician receives a patient with a minimum of tasks done, namely the registration and the vitals. The MA accompanies the patient into the room where the doctor takes the history and does the physical. The MA enters the information into the EMR.

SCRIBING A VERBALLY TAKEN history into a written EMR requires solid familiarity with the EMR. The MA must know which points belong in the gyn section, which in ob, which in medical, and which in the surgical section. Medications and allergies can be reviewed in advance after vitals, or can be done in concert with the history.

. . .

SCRIBING MUST BE DONE by someone who is a quick typist. A scribe must also have a good grasp of spelling and grammar. Finally, she must be fluent in medical terminology.

THE SCRIBE MUST UNDERSTAND her EMR (Electronic Medical Record) document. She must know just where everything goes. EMRs vary in structure, but most have templates to be filled, boxes to click and selected areas for free text. With familiarity, these can be filled quickly, even if the history narrative twists and turns.

IT IS, of course, helpful if the doctor does not let the history twist and turn too much. Traditionally, a history has a prescribed flow. Medical students of a certain age were all taught roughly the same thing as detailed above. Before asking an MA to scribe, the physician directors or senior staff should train MAs in this traditional history taking.

AFTER THE HISTORY, the doctor moves on to the physical examination. One advantage of the scribing system is that it provides for a built in chaperone. It also provides for a built in assistant if cultures or other specimens need to be taken. Sometimes, when packages or jars need to be opened, it is good to have an extra pair of hands. Certainly, if any office procedures need to be done, an assistant is essential.

AFTER THE HISTORY AND PHYSICAL, the doctor establishes a differential diagnosis and discusses her assessment and plans. The scribe fills the predetermined section in the EMR in real time, and orders are placed on the spot. By the time the patient is ready to leave the room, the documentation and orders are done.

SCRIBING HAS ITS ADVANTAGES. Patients and staff wait less for orders, scripts, and follow up to be put into the system. There is less down time between patients. The doctor spends more time doctoring.

THE DOWNSIDE of the scribing system is that it requires a higher degree of training than that required from an MA who simply performs vital signs and rooms the patient. That downside, however, leads to another set of upsides. The medical assistant who can scribe gets to know her patients better. She gets to learn history taking from her physician partner. She gets that much more familiar with the process of medicine since she hears the discussion of the medical assessment and the rationale behind the plans as explained to the patient. An MA who can scribe becomes an excellent phone triage person, and better at explaining things to patients.

THE SCRIBE METHOD does not require an MA to work her way through a complicated medical history without the benefit of the physician by her side. With scribing, the time-consuming part of the visit is only done once. The doctor, patient, and MA all get done sooner. As a bonus, the front will have their orders the minute the patient comes to check out.

. . .

A HYBRID APPROACH can be employed. It is possible to begin with conventional utilization of the medical assistant. If at any point the physician needs help with a physical exam, an unplanned procedure, a chaperone, or order entry, she can simply ask the MA to step-in. This has the potential to disrupt the MA's workflow, so physicians should use this strategy mindfully. If, at the onset of the visit, either the MA or the physician senses the visit will be challenging, they should check in with one another in case they could use help.

THESE POINTS about scribing may soon become moot. These days, a staffing shortage is at hand. Scribing may become a luxury.

MEDICAL ASSISTANT CHARTING has to be as professional as anyone else's. MAs like nurses or doctors have to find that balance between brevity and completeness in their charting.

MEDICAL DOCUMENTATION NOTES should be written with a few people in mind: a future caregiver trying to make sense out of the patient's condition, an attorney trying to discern whether malpractice took place, and the patient herself reading the medical record.

NOTES SHOULD STAY professional and factual. The chart should not contain editorials or arguments over care between caregivers.

.   .   .

ONE EASY WAY TO keep documentation quality high is to complete it in a timely fashion. Those of us who have done this for a while will tell you it is not a good idea to leave charts for later. Always finish charting as soon as you can after the care is rendered. Your notes will be more accurate and you will feel more relaxed and satisfied.

IN ALL CASES, the caregiver must review and clarify all that the MA has recorded. *History taking is an art and comes with experience and relationship with the patient.*

IT IS WELL KNOWN that patients sometimes give a different history to different caregivers. This is a phenomenon that medical students and residents call "scooping". When the patient tells the resident more than he tells the medical student, that medical student has "been scooped". Those getting scooped should not take it personally.

THE WAY MAs and physicians collaborate depends on the practice type, practice volume, staffing availability, and the individual caregivers themselves. There is an infinity of ways to do it well. Hopefully, by highlighting all the components of the process, a dynamic custom approach can be crafted for each unique practice.

INTRODUCTION TO PROCEDURES

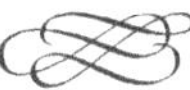

It is no wonder that coming in for an annual examination is anxiety producing. After all, you are coming in to be stripped down, poked and prodded, sampled and scanned, so that trained professionals have the highest possible chance of finding something wrong with you.

MOST OF THE TIME, something bad is not found. However, something questionable may be. In offices which care for women, abnormalities are often investigated by procedures. Obstetrics and gynecology is an evidence-based and rather quantitative profession. We prefer definitive diagnoses. These are often obtained by blood tests and tissue samples. Those are obtained through procedures.

SOME OF THESE procedures are more invasive than others. Because of this, the patient's anxiety is at least threefold compared to an ordinary doctor's visit. First, she might be concerned about the physical discomfort of the procedure. Second, she might be concerned about the cost. Not only is the procedure done by a trained professional who requires reimbursement, it is handled and processed in a different facility, often a laboratory or hospital. Each generate separate bills. Finally, she is concerned about the results.

THE MEDICAL ASSISTANT is wise to be aware of all these sources of anxiety. In most cases, patient's expectations about procedures are worse than the procedure itself. Over time, the experienced medical assistant can see this for herself. When she informs a patient that a procedure will be necessary, she can share her experience. She can remind the patient that many before her have had procedures done, and lived to go shopping shortly thereafter.

THE FRONT OFFICE has a role in calming patient anxiety. Well before the procedure, staff should go over all the procedure's associated costs, as best can be determined. The staff should be clear about the tolerances of their estimate. This means they should give a margin of error on both low and high sides of their estimate. ***Patients can plan and do best psychologically if they are given realistic information.***

DOING procedures well begins long before the patient arrives. First, the provider and the medical assistant must have the requisite skill set. With technology advancing every year, new techniques and new equipment come along to improve our procedures and make our results more accurate. Caregivers must remain current with all the certification and training that such new technology requires. They can pass their knowledge on to their medical assistants who help with these procedures.

Providers should appreciate that medical assistants should never be thrown into assisting with a procedure until they are adequately trained. *Providers and patients should recognize that there is nothing wrong with having two medical assistants in the room, one learning and the other assisting.*

While procedures are often done in the office of an obstetrician gynecologist, the procedure types are limited. The variety in a week can be counted on two hands, if not one. That said, *there is something unique about each patient's procedure.* The most common procedures are colposcopy, endometrial biopsy, intrauterine device (IUD) insertion and IUD removal. Less common are perineal skin biopsy, Nexplanon insertion and Nexplanon removal.

Regardless of the test or procedure, the patient should have the indication for the procedure clear in her mind. This falls to both the medical assistant and the doctor. At the appointment when the procedure is planned, the caregiver should make sure that the patient understands her diagnosis. She should also understand why that diagnosis merits a certain procedure. The procedure itself should be described, including how it is done. Risks, benefits, complications and alternatives to that procedure should be discussed. This discussion is the basis of consent.

. . .

CAREGIVERS SHOULD DISCUSS THE "DIFFERENTIAL DIAGNOSIS". The differential diagnosis is the list of possible diagnoses that the procedure could reveal. It is the answer to the inevitable question, "What could it be?"

IT IS tricky to discuss differential diagnosis without further provoking the patient's anxiety. The reason for this is that the differential diagnosis can often go from the entirely benign to the sinister. The key to discussing the differential diagnosis is putting matters into context and perspective. It is helpful to remind the patient that benign diseases are common and that serious ones are less common.

WHEN THE PATIENT is scheduled for a procedure and a complex differential diagnosis is under consideration the patient should be reminded that medicine is inherently conservative. While we believe that most of the time most everything is okay, we also believe in pursuing that small chance that something is not okay. Why? So we can treat it.

CHANCES ARE, the patient has undergone a screening test. The Pap is an example of a screening test. The Pap itself and the interpretations of Pap smears are purposefully designed to over diagnose. Because of this, they are unlikely to miss anything bad. The "price" for this sensitivity is a tendency to report as abnormal that which is actually normal. Said another way, screening tests like the pap are designed to be very sensitive, but not very specific.

.   .   .

IT IS the policy of medicine to use screening tests which have this heightened sensitivity. We do this across the board with not only Pap smears but studies like mammograms and blood tests.

*AS A GROUP OF PROFESSIONALS, **we are loath to miss a diagnosis. We are trained, psychologically and technically, to find and fix problems. We are driven to fix things while they are treatable, well before they progress and become untreatable.***

IF PATIENTS UNDERSTOOD THIS, they might forgive us for all the times when expensive, uncomfortable procedures returned normal results.

PAPERWORK HELPS WITH THIS PROCESS. The medical assistant can give the patient a handout about the procedure. This explains how to prepare, what to expect, reasons to call the office afterwards, and the follow up.

PAPERWORK CAN BE GIVEN as paper or it can be a link to a website with the same content. Either way, the chart needs to show that the patient was given this information. I can think of at least one lawsuit that hinged on the documentation of this sheet being given.

A PRE-PROCEDURE INFORMATION sheet for colposcopy might include a brief paragraph about the pathophysiology of human papillomavirus and a refresher about the Pap itself. The sheet can also include information about how the procedure is done. For example, patients might be reassured to know it is similar to a pap smear, but uses a magnification light called a colposcope. They might also appreciate that the biopsies taken are tiny, perhaps smaller than half a split pea. The sheet may include instructions to take Tylenol or ibuprofen half an hour before the procedure. It must include specific warning signs such as fever for which the doctor must be called.

Even if patients are told about procedures, chances are, they will remember imperfectly. I will periodically reiterate that *the smartest patient paying the most attention takes home only half of what we say.* Therefore, in my office, we refer them to a page on our website which is pertinent to their procedure, so that they can review what they were told in the comfort of their home. We ask them to read over the information when they get home and invite them to search on the internet if they want to with, of course, a caveat.

When patients consult the internet, it is crucial that they be mindful of the source. There is no better way for a patient to scare themself than to read on some unmonitored message board.

Sometimes I draw diagrams or make sticky notes and give them to the patient. I also ask them to take pictures of them with their smartphone. This way, I know the information cannot get lost.

.   .   .

ANXIETY LEVELS GO DOWN if a person is well rested. It is worth reminding patients to eat properly, exercise and have good sleep hygiene in the days prior to a procedure, especially the night before. However, sometimes the procedure provokes so much anxiety that good sleep is not possible. If the patient anticipates this will be the case, an anxiolytic or sleep medication can be prescribed.

CERTAIN PROCEDURES warrant pre-procedure acetaminophen and or ibuprofen. If a patient is especially anxious, she can receive an anxiolytic medication like Ativan 30 to 45 minutes prior to procedure, provided that she has someone to bring her and take her home.

WE HAVE ALREADY DISCUSSED the inherent conservatism of screening tests and touched upon the metrics of sensitivity and specificity. One way to express this to a nervous patient is by reminding them that **horses are more common than zebras.** In this proverb, horses are benign common conditions, and zebras are rare sinister ones. This is an image that should stick in their minds, even if they are anxious.

THIS REITERATES our earlier key point. It means that most likely something benign, self-limited or manageable will be diagnosed. If something unusual, exotic or concerning (a zebra) is found, it is our chance to do something effective about it. Said another way, knowledge is power. *Knowledge is still power, even if the knowledge is concerning.*

.   .   .

AT THIS STAGE, before we go into the details of different procedures, a general piece of advice is warranted. Procedures are a little like cooking, French cooking, to be exact. French cooking is known for its precision and for its disregard of simplicity. Before you know it, you've used every dish in the kitchen.

PROCEDURES CAN BE LIKE THIS. Preparation is essential. In French cooking, this strategy is called "mise en place", literally, to put in place. In cooking, it includes three steps. First is to read the recipe from start to finish. Second, is to assemble all the ingredients and equipment necessary to prepare the recipe. Third, it means completing as many steps as you can before the actual mixing, such as measuring out the ingredients into prep bowls.

AS APPLIED to medicine and surgery, the first step is reviewing the chart for the indications of the procedure. Second, it means checking and assembling all the requisite equipment. Third, it means getting whatever possible done in advance, such as pulling the necessary medications and arranging the equipment on a mayo stand.

YOU SHOULD HAVE A FULLY STOCKED instrument cart on wheels that's easy to move, that will fit in the room, that goes with you for every single procedure, no matter how simple or low risk it may seem at first. You must also let your fellow staff members know you are going in for a procedure. In this way, they can avoid sending spurious or interruptive calls to you and they can be listening if you call out for their help.

· · ·

Many procedures cannot be done if the patient is pregnant. Preparation for these procedures therefore requires a sound determination that the patient is not pregnant. This is especially important for any procedures that broach the intrauterine cavity or the endocervical canal. Final determination that the patient is not pregnant depends on history plus a urine or blood pregnancy test. The final decision rests with the physician who will perform the procedure, but the MA must also have this question firmly in her mind.

Small invasive procedures are a routine part of the functioning of a gynecology office. These procedures are critical to patient care. They are also a lot of fun.

You might ask, how can something medically important and potentially uncomfortable for the patient possibly be fun for the caregiver? The answer lies in skill. We experience a sense of fun if we can do something necessary for which we are well prepared. There is also a sense of accomplishment in doing things that unequivocally need doing. The real satisfaction comes in doing it well.

COLPOSCOPY (COLPO)

Colposcopy is simply an examination with a colposcope. A colposcope is simply a set of magnification lenses with a bright light and a green filter. When a pap smear comes back abnormal, we need a better examination of the cervix. We use the enhanced vision of the colposcope to direct the location of our biopsies. This makes our results much more accurate. Biopsy based results are both more sensitive and more specific.

THE PAP SMEAR is a routine cancer screening test. It is indicated on women over 21 years of age. It tests for cancers caused by the human papillomavirus, or HPV for short. HPV can cause cancer because it is made largely of DNA. It inserts its DNA into the DNA of our own cervical cells. Since DNA provides instructions for the cell's growth and development, the abnormal viral DNA instructs the cells to grow abnormally, creating pre-cancerous and cancerous changes in the epithelium of the cervix. It is a relatively slow process from virus to cancer. Therefore, with regular screening, we can detect and interrupt these cancer-causing processes. The Pap smear is that screening.

THE PAP SMEAR consists of brushing a soft small plastic brush on the cervix. This collects loose cells not only from the surface of the cervix but also from the distal endocervical canal. The brush is swished in a jar of formalin and sent to the laboratory for analysis.

THIS IS NOT A VERY refined method of assessing the cells on the cervix. It's just a sample of detached cells and the sampling does not go deep. The technicians and the machines that read the specimen can only go so far in their analyses. With only a Pap smear, it is only possible to discern four broad categories: normal, atypical cells, low-grade changes, and high-grade changes. This is insufficient to guide therapy, but it is enough to tell us if biopsies are needed.

. . .

To determine whether to pursue further studies beyond the Pap, several things are taken into consideration. Principal among them is the HPV status, which is tested by PCR (polymerase chain reaction), a very sensitive assay. Next is the pap reading itself, the patient's age, whether the patient is pregnant and their risk factors. Factoring in all these variables is so complex that an app has been provided for us by the ASCCP, the Association of Cervical Colposcopists and Pathologists, the governing organization for these protocols. Yes, "there's an app for that."

Assuming the protocol indicates further studies are necessary, a colposcopy is performed. With Pap smears we obtain detached cells, whereas, with colposcopy we obtain chunks of cells. These chunks are no bigger than half of a split pea, but they reveal a great deal more than a simple smear. In particular, they reveal the architecture of the tissue layer. We can see the relationship of the cells to one another. Normally, they should be organized in a certain way. However, if human papillomavirus is present in the tissues and the instructions for the cells' behavior have been corrupted by the virus, the cell layers may be disorganized in a characteristic way. We can recognize these changes in the chunks of tissue obtained by colposcopy.

It is important to be careful when choosing words to describe these procedures to patients. For example, the word "chunk" is somewhat misleading. Sometimes the biopsies from colposcopy are so tiny that we can scarcely see them as they float in a jar of formalin. When discussing a prospective procedure with the patient, mindful language should always be used. Informing a patient about the details of a procedure beforehand is a best practice, but the devil is in the details.

COLPOSCOPY IS PRINCIPALLY AN EXAMINATION. The colposcope is nothing more than an ordinary bright light with magnification and color filters. For the abnormal tissues to show up the best, we first apply vinegar and then, barring an allergy, an iodine containing solution. Before applying, we should routinely ask patients if they are allergic to iodine or shellfish which contain iodine. We then examine and identify areas which may appear concerning. The Lugol's solution penetrates normal squamous epithelium on the cervix, making it dark blackish blue. However, if there is dysplasia or abnormal cell growth on the cervix, that region turns white. We call it a "nonstaining region". This is where the gynecologist should biopsy in order to get the highest yield to find the worst dysplasia.

WHEN THE BIOPSY IS TAKEN, the doctor should tell the medical assistant where it was taken from. We describe the surface of the cervix like we do the face of a clock. We identify the location of the biopsy by "time", i.e six o'clock. Commonly, up to four biopsies are needed. Each of these requires a separate labeled jar. We use an instrument with a tiny cutter to obtain a sample from the surface of the cervix. Sometimes these specimens are difficult to remove from the instrument. The sharp end of a broken wooden q tip may help tease it out.

. . .

AT THAT POINT, unless the patient is pregnant, we use an endocervical curette to take a specimen from the endocervical canal. This feels a little crampy, but again, only for a few seconds. This specimen goes in a separate jar. I like to take the endocervical curette with the specimen and swish it into a formalin jar until the specimen comes off into the liquid. In this way, we get a full assessment of the cells of the cervix.

THE MEDICAL ASSISTANT must take care of all the specimens, labelling them correctly. She may also have to help the doctor and make sure that the patient is hemostatic. There is usually a little bleeding from the biopsy sites. Most of the time, a couple minutes of pressure is all that is necessary to stop the bleeding. This can be done with a regular Q-Tip or even a sponge on a stick. A sponge on a stick is a ring forceps with a tightly folded gauze 4 x 4 between the tongs. Occasionally, a silver nitrate stick is necessary to chemically cauterize the bleeding biopsy site.

AFTER ALL THE biopsies are taken, the patient should continue to rest supine for 5 to 10 minutes. She should get up only with the supervision of the medical assistant. This is regardless of how the patient feels.

PATIENTS CANNOT ALWAYS PREDICT if they are going to be lightheaded after a procedure. They will feel fine until the second that they don't.

REACTIONS of this nature are called vagal or vasovagal reactions. They are unpredictable and are usually delayed by five minutes. It is a response that is hard wired deeply into the subcortical regions of the brain. It has nothing to do with "toughness" or "will power".

AFTERWARDS, patients may expect a watery or blood tinged vaginal discharge. Spotting is a normal part of healing. The discharge may also contain a brownish material which comes from the medication apply to the cervix. Patient should put nothing in the vagina, including tampons, douching or intercourse until the spotting stops, which may take up to seven days.

PATIENTS ARE to call in with the following criteria:

1. Fever, chills, nausea or vomiting.
2. Vaginal bleeding more than spotting.
3. Pain worse than menstrual cramps.
4. Foul discharge.

Remind the patient that the results will be back in about five business days. If they do not hear back, they should call.

IMMEDIATELY AFTER COLPOSCOPY, patients are typically eager to discuss their plan. They should be gently reminded that their care plan will be based on the results of the colposcopy, so that discussion will have to wait until results return.

ENDOMETRIAL BIOPSY (EMB)

Patients often confuse biopsies of the cervix with biopsies of the endometrium. The endometrium is the lining of the uterus. The uterus is a pear-shaped organ which sits at the top of the vagina. The small end is called the cervix and the large end is called the fundus. The uterine wall is made of muscle, but the lining, the endometrium, is glandular. It is the source of our period and the normal location of implantation of a pregnancy.

THE CERVIX IS JUST the end of the uterus, but its surface and its lining are histologically distinct from the rest of the uterus and the endometrium. This means that the cells are different. They are so different that they are subject to different disease processes. As mentioned above, the cells of the cervix and endocervix are vulnerable to disease caused by the human papillomavirus.

THE ENDOMETRIUM IS HORMONALLY sensitive and swells and evacuates every month during normal menstruation. However, the system can go awry. Hormonally mediated changes can occur in these cells, causing them to become pre-cancerous or cancerous. This type of change is usually manifested by abnormal uterine bleeding. Such abnormal bleeding requires investigation, especially if it occurs during certain circumstances or in patients with certain risk factors, such as menopause. Those with abnormal bleeding who are older, or who have risk factors for endometrial disease are candidates for biopsy. These risk factors include hypertension, diabetes, and obesity. They can also include a positive family history of uterine cancer.

THE PATIENT SHOULD UNDERSTAND her risk factors for endometrial disease and her indications for the procedure.

She should understand the risks, benefits, complications, and alternatives (RBCA) and have signed a consent. The procedure has minor risks of causing bleeding, infection, disturbing a pregnancy, or perforation of the uterine wall. These risks are rare and the benefits of the procedure are high. Hopefully, the doctor explains these things, but it is good for the MA to have this knowledge as well.

ABNORMAL BLEEDING CAN TAKE the form of menorrhagia, which is regular periods which are unusually heavy or long. Menometrorrhagia is also an indication for an endometrial biopsy. This condition consists of periods that are deranged in both flow and timing. Finally, endometrial biopsy is indicated if imaging reveals an abnormal endometrial appearance, i.e. when it is unduly thickened, irregular or cystic.

TO SET up for endometrial biopsy is a little more complicated than to setup for colposcopy. That is because endometrial biopsy potentially requires a wider variety of instruments.

ENDOMETRIAL BIOPSY INVOLVES SLIDING a thin plunger equipped tube up through the cervix and into the full depth of the uterus. These tubes go by various brand names.

ANYTHING like this that touches the muscle wall of the uterus will create a cramp. This is because the uterus is a muscle and will contract upon being touched. Tylenol (acetaminophen) or ibuprofen could be given half hour beforehand, but it is unclear how much benefit this would confer on such a brief procedure.

As with all procedures, I feel it is most prudent to bring in the whole mobile surgical cart. The procedure is a sterile procedure. Therefore, a mayo stand with a sterile drape should also be prepared. Sterile instruments should be available but not necessarily unpackaged.

Before an endometrial biopsy is done, a bimanual exam is performed so that the doctor can determine the uterine size and directionality. This is necessary since it can provide guidance on how to slide instruments into the uterus. Without knowing the shape and length of the interior cavity of the uterus, the doctor can perforate the uterus.

We call this measurement "sounding" the uterus. We use a thin malleable rod called a uterine sound. This instrument has a blunt end to help prevent perforation. It is marked in centimeters so that the doctor will know how far to insert the Pipelle, the biopsy straw. If the uterine sound cannot be introduced, the anterior lip of the cervix should be numbed either with a freeze spray or some lidocaine. The single toothed tenaculum is used to grasp the anterior lip of the cervix. Often, with a little traction on the anterior lip of the cervix, the sound can be introduced. If not, the cervix may be dilated, and the sound tried again. Once in a while, the Pipelle itself is the best dilator since it is a little smaller than the sound.

. . .

ONCE ENTRY IS GAINED, the Pipelle is swished around inside the endometrial cavity, collecting the specimen as a doctor withdraws the interior rod of the Pipelle, creating suction. This is typically when the patient feels her worst cramps. The patient should be encouraged to breathe for relaxation, and reminded that the procedure only lasts a few seconds. Once withdrawn, the cramp should stop. In a few minutes, even the dull ache should pass.

WHILE THE PATIENT rests on the table, the doctor presents the Pipelle with the specimen to the medical assistant. The MA has a specimen jar ready. She positions the open specimen jar underneath the Pipelle, often on the mayo stand, and uses scissors to snip off the end. The doctor then plunges the specimen into the formalin inside the jar. The clear formalin permits a visual assessment of the amount of specimen in the jar. If there is not enough, more should be obtained.

THE MA LABELS the container in the room, since her primary responsibility at this stage is to watch the patient. As with all procedures, the patient needs to be watched for a few minutes, even if they are feeling fine. Most people do well afterwards and carry on with their normal day.

IF SOMETHING ABNORMAL IS FOUND, it is worth remembering that endometrial pathologies are some of the most treatable conditions in gynecology. There is a very low threshold to perform an endometrial biopsy. Said another way, there's very little downside to performing an endometrial biopsy compared to the enormous benefits that it can confer. The various diseases that can arise in the endometrium are, like most other diseases, best treated when they are diagnosed and treated as early as possible.

THE MA IS USUALLY in charge of giving the patients her aftercare instructions and precautions. For endometrial biopsy, they are as follows:

AFTER THE PROCEDURE:

1. You may have mild cramping over the next 24 hours, but it should gradually subside.
2. Depending on the phase of your cycle when you were biopsied, you will have vaginal bleeding, which should not exceed that of a medium period, or last for more than a week.

Instructions:

1. No intercourse, douching or tampons for at least 48 hours.
2. Resume other normal activities as soon as you feel able.
3. Bathing by tub or shower is acceptable.

Notify us regarding any of the following:

1. Fever, chills, nausea or vomiting.
2. Vaginal bleeding greater than a moderate period or greater than one pad per hour.
3. Foul vaginal discharge.
4. Pain worse than menstrual cramps.

Patients should know that results will be available within about five working days or sooner. Patients should be encouraged to call if they do not hear back.

CERVICAL POLYPECTOMY

Cervical polyps are common, occurring in women of reproductive age and sometimes later. They are basically a glandular outgrowth of cells from the endocervical canal. It is unclear why they arise. Cervical polyps are almost always benign. Why do we consistently want to remove them when we find them? The reasons are several. First, they can interfere with the Pap smear. Second, they grow and can cause spotting. They can get infected.

CERVICAL POLYPECTOMY IS SIMPLER than the aforementioned procedures such as colposcopy. However, it is a procedure, so a consent form is necessary. It can cause uterine cramping, so the hot pack is beneficial.

POLYPS ARE USUALLY NOTICED at the time of the routine Pap smear, since most of the time they are small and asymptomatic. During the reproductive years, their natural history is to grow and sometimes avulse spontaneously.

WHEN THEY ARE LARGER, they are more likely to produce symptoms such as mid-cycle bleeding or ongoing discharge. These signs may mean the polyp is infected. Any time there is a concurrent vaginitis or cervicitis at the time of discovery, the infection should be treated before an attempted removal.

The medical assistant should reinforce the doctor's decision to wait for removal. This leaves some patients frustrated because once a lesion is discovered, they want it promptly removed.

THE TECHNIQUE of cervical polyp removal depends on the size of the polyp. It also depends on the shape of the polyp. Though the procedure is small, it is prudent to begin with cleansing the area with Betadine or Hibiclens, and to use a bit of freeze spray not only for analgesia, but also for vaso-constriction. If the polyp is bulbous and on a small stalk, it is a simple matter to grasp the polyp with a ring forceps, twist the polyp off the stalk, which renders the severed stalk hemostatic. Usually, no additional hemostatic agents or procedures are necessary. However, as with other procedures, it is prudent to have the surgical cart in the room in case a stitch is necessary. It is also useful to have silver nitrate available for chemical cautery.

IN THE OPERATING ROOM, when I have medical students, residents, nursing students, and even seasoned nurses, I like them to visualize the procedure themselves before assisting with it. This helps because they should be at least one step ahead of me. This is true not only for hospital-based surgeries but also for clinic based procedures. That is why I go into particular detail here, so that the medical assistant can know what is going on beyond her view and beyond the present moment.

ON THAT NOTE, it is good for the medical assistant to see what is going on from the doctor's standpoint. Periodically, the doctor should pause the procedure and ask the MA to have a look so that she gains perspective and experience.

PATIENTS UNDERGOING polypectomy should be told from the beginning that can be a multistage procedure. Sometimes just the top of the polyp is removed, and a dangling bit of the base is left behind. That is why polypectomy patients should have a follow-up visit sometime around one to two weeks post procedure to check healing and to see if any polyp remains.

PATIENTS SHOULD ALSO KNOW that during the reproductive years, polyps have a tendency to grow back, even if they were entirely removed. They are an estrogen dependent entity and can regrow in the reproductive years when estrogen is plentiful.

A FIRST TIME premenopausal polyp does not necessarily need to be sent to pathology if it is of average size and appearance. If the polyp taken represents a recurrence, it should be sent to pathology.

POLYPS CAN APPEAR in the post-menopausal period as well. When they do, the index of concern is higher. The removal needs to be more complete, and the specimen needs to be sent to pathology.

ONCE IN A WHILE, a polyp is too large to be removed in the clinic. Its stalk may appear to be thick or beyond where the doctor can see, in the endocervical canal or the uterus. These cases are best done in the operating room, where pain control, exposure and instrumentation are optimized.

PERINEAL BIOPSY

The perineal biopsy is not as invasive as an endometrial biopsy or an IUD insertion. Nonetheless, it can be more painful. This is because the perineal tissue is densely innervated. Therefore, we use anesthetic in this procedure.

PIGMENTED lesions of the vulva and perineum deserve biopsy. Examples would be dense white areas, raised bumps, and dark variegated spots. The differential diagnosis of these lesions ranges from HPV mediated disease such as condyloma, to vulvar intraepithelial neoplasia (VIN), lichen sclerosis, or melanoma.

To BEGIN, as always, the procedure is explained and consent is signed. A hot pad may be comforting. If the patient is in menopause experiencing hot flashes, this may not be the case. Skin is initially prepped. After that, we apply freeze spray in anticipation of the injection of a local anesthetic. At that point, pressure is applied, and adequate time is given for the anesthetic to take effect. The right instrument is chosen. It can range from a Tischler ectocervical biopsy forcep to a scalpel or even small scissors with pickups with teeth.

This brings me to the general issue of instruments. All the MAs should know the names of all the instruments. There should be a consensus among the medical assistants on where instruments are stored, so that in the event of urgent need, any of the MAs can find any of the instruments quickly. In our office, we have a surgical instrument cart which can be rolled around easily as needed. It has multiple small drawers. Once a consensus is achieved about where certain instruments go, the drawers can be labeled.

Instruments are chosen based on the size and location of the lesion. Lesions can form on the labia minora, including the clitoral hood, and the perineum, the space between the posterior opening of the vagina and rectum. The former tissue is delicate, and the latter is tougher, making instrument selection custom. In procedures such as this, the MA needs to be ready for anything.

MOST OF THE TIME, perineal biopsies bleed. Biopsy sites can be made hemostatic with small stitches or silver nitrate cautery sticks. Occasionally, pressure and Steri-Strips will do the trick, though these will not stay put.

POST PROCEDURE CARE INCLUDES "SITS" baths, which is really just a bath in a clean tub with plain water. These need to be done fairly frequently at first: two times a day, if not three. As the site heals, that frequency can be decreased to daily if the site is not prone to discharge. The patient should call in right away if the lesion becomes increasingly painful, puffy or produces any purulent fluid.

IT SEEMS like endometrial and cervical biopsies are relatively self sterilizing in a way that perineal biopsies are not. This is likely from their exposure to the environment, specifically skin flora. The patient should check her site daily until it is healed. The medical assistant can reinforce these messages to the patient as she gets her ready to leave the clinic. As always, the patient should leave the clinic with post procedure instructions. The procedure note should document that this is the case.

IUD INSERTION AND REMOVAL

IUD insertion is a common procedure, and shares certain features in common with endometrial biopsy. This is because we have to slide something through the cervical canal and into the endometrial cavity. For endometrial biopsy, IUD insertion, and really any procedure where cramping or discomfort is expected, a warm pack should be prepared for the patient. These can be commercial or homemade rice or buckwheat bags, as long as they are cleanable, or covered with a disposable or washable drape. The warmth seems to reduce uterine cramping.

FOR PROCEDURES that do not actually produce uterine cramping, warm packs still provide comfort and relaxation. This is especially true if the bag is treated with a few drops of essential oil prior to being heated in the microwave. We recommend lavender oil, because it is such a favorite, but also citrus oils including lemon, lime, orange, and grapefruit. The citrus essential oils, in particular, have been shown to enhance mood.

ONCE THE HOT pack has been placed and the paperwork has been signed, the procedure is similar to an endometrial biopsy. A bimanual exam is performed, and a speculum is placed. The cervix is cleansed, sounded, dilated if need be, and the IUD is inserted. The doctor will then request a pair of scissors because the IUD's string will be cut to a convenient length. The patient is then observed per protocol.

IUD REMOVAL IS USUALLY a simple matter. They are rarely stuck. If they are, the vast majority of them can be removed in clinic with a little endocervical exploration. If IUD removal consists of anything but the usual gentle pull of the string, then the Medical Assistant should be asked to bring the hot pack, the surgical cart, and a general consent form. The patient is prepped with betadine before instruments are inserted up the endocervical canal. The degree to which this is necessary varies per situation. Sometimes a plastic endocervical brush is all that is needed to tease the IUD string out into a reachable place. Sometimes dilation and a polyp forceps are needed.

ANY PROCEDURE such as this which causes the patient undue discomfort should be aborted and resumed in the surgical suite. If this is planned, the patient should be informed about the change in costs. She will be grateful for the new information.

POST PROCEDURE

All procedures, no matter how simple or small, have the potential for reactions and side effects. Patients should know this from the onset, but this caution should be tempered with the reality that, in the vast majority of cases, procedures go well with no complications.

· · ·

THE MOST IMMEDIATE post procedure complication is pain or tenderness. Office procedures are chosen explicitly because they have mild or temporary pain. These discomforts have usually passed by the time the patient leaves the office, if not sooner.

THE NEXT MOST IMMEDIATE potential complication is the previously mentioned vasovagal reaction. A vagal reaction is a sudden slowing of the heart rate caused by activation of the vagus nerve, which slows down the heart rate as a part of the body's natural response to pain or stress. However, the reaction can occasionally be excessive. The heart rate can drop too far, resulting in under perfusion of the brain, and the patient faints. This also means that they collapse, and potentially hurt themself.

OFTEN, the fainting is preceded by a sense of lightheadedness and or nausea. Sometimes there is no warning. The MA should always be alert for this possibility, even if there is no past history of it. Patients should be watched five minutes after the procedure since the reaction is sometimes delayed.

THE PATIENT SHOULD LEAVE the office with information about what was done, what was seen, if anything, the post procedure expectations, limitations of activity and any precautions for which she must call in. Ideally, this all comes in a one-page handout or a web link. A follow-up visit should be scheduled. She should be given a rough idea of when results are to be expected.

MEDICAL ASSISTANT
PROCEDURES

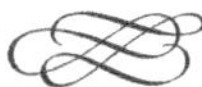

It makes sense that the trained medical assistant can perform certain procedures on her own. Phlebotomy, injections and urine catheterization are good examples.

PHLEBOTOMY

Phlebotomy is the process of collecting blood samples for laboratory testing. The following steps outline the basic procedure for performing phlebotomy.

1. Prepare the equipment: Gather necessary supplies, including a sterile needle, tourniquet, alcohol pads, gauze, and a collection vial.
2. Identify the patient. Verify the patient's identity and the correct site for the blood draw.
3. Clean the chosen venipuncture site with an alcohol pad to prevent infection.

4. Apply the tourniquet: Apply the tourniquet above the site to locate a vein and make it more prominent.
5. Locate the vein: Palpate the vein to locate it and position the needle at a 15 to 30-degree angle with respect to the skin.
6. Insert the needle: Quickly insert the needle into the vein and attach the tubing to the needle. When you are in the vein securely, loosen the tourniquet.
7. Collect the sample: Fill the collection vial with the required amount of blood.
8. After the collection is complete, remove the needle and place pressure on the site with gauze to assist with clotting and prevent bruising.
9. Safely dispose of the needle in a sharps box.
10. Label the sample with the patient's name, date and time of draw.

NOTE: This is a basic outline. Specific techniques and procedures may vary depending on the training and protocols of the facility or organization.

NOW FOR THE rest of the story. There are many tips and tricks for getting blood from a patient. There are many reasons blood can be difficult to get out of patients. The patient may have small veins. She may have veins which roll. On the other side of the spectrum, the patient may be very heavy. Her subcutaneous tissues may obscure the location or sensation of her veins. Finally, and most commonly, patients may be dehydrated. This might be because they are ill, or it might be because we have asked them to have nothing to eat or drink for eight hours before their blood draw. They may forget that this does not include water.

IN THESE PATIENTS, several maneuvers may be helpful. First, you can make sure that they wear any coat that they may have brought or do whatever they have to do to get as warm as possible. You can give them a glass of hot water to drink. A hot pack can be applied to the site. These measures are to get them to vasodilate.

YOU CAN SETTLE them into a chair or onto a table with a tourniquet around their arm with the arm placed lower than their heart. Of course, lighting should be optimized. Usually, these measures are more than enough to make the blood draw possible.

PHLEBOTOMY SHOULD ONLY BE PERFORMED by trained medical professionals with certification. That said, all but four states do not require any phlebotomy certification or license to draw blood. However, even in states with no requirements, it is best to have an in clinic-based certification and sign off procedure. Even better, the candidate should complete some sort of online didactic training and in-house practicum with an experienced member of the staff.

IN CLINIC LAB draws can be a great convenience for patients who do not want to navigate the bigger setting of the hospital environment. However, there are some downsides. Phlebotomy does not reimburse much, and it takes the medical assistant away from other patient care duties. Every office is going to have to decide whether clinic phlebotomy makes sense for them.

URINE CATHETERIZATIONS

Physicians often perform urine catheterization in the course of a pelvic exam. In our clinic, established patients have drop-in rights for a few conditions, like possible urinary tract infection. The average patient can get by with a clean catch. However, anyone suspected of being unable to perform a good clean catch should have a catheterization. People in this category include the pregnant, those with large abdominal girth, the young, or the very elderly.

CAUTION SHOULD BE EXERCISED in choosing patients for a urine catheterization. Some find it fairly uncomfortable, so the risk-benefit ratio should be carefully assessed. Children should get a catheterization only if absolutely necessary.

THE FOLLOWING steps outline the basic procedure of urinary catheterization.

1. Prepare the equipment: Gather the equipment, such as a sterile catheter, gloves, sterile lubricant, and a collection container.
2. Explain the procedure to the patient: Explain what will happen and why it is being done.
3. Wash your hands: Do this thoroughly with soap and water for at least fifteen seconds.
4. Don the gloves.

5. Place the patient in stirrups and locate the urethral opening. This is at the anterior aspect of the vagina in women.
6. Apply a small amount of lubricant to the end of the catheter.
7. Slowly insert the catheter, advancing until urine flows.
8. Collect the specimen into the tube.
9. Remove the catheter, taking care not to touch the catheter or the specimen.
10. Dispose of the equipment properly and wash your hands again.

I HAVE FOUND it useful to ask the patient to take a couple of full breaths. Then, I ask them to exhale with force. At that moment, I insert the catheter. This seems to minimize distress with the procedure. Oddly, removal seems to be as annoying as the insertion, so we use the same technique.

INJECTIONS

Injections, while simple, are not without risk. Following a consistent protocol, together with sensitivity to specific patient's risk factors, will minimize these risks.

UNDERSTANDING a patient's risk factors is a matter of being familiar with their medical history. Long before they are receiving injections in the office, their medical history should be clearly documented in the clinic chart. The MA just needs to read it. And, in greeting the patient for the visit, the MA should ask if there have been any issues with injections in the past. These are things that the chart might not reflect and that the doctor might not know.

REACTIONS TO INJECTIONS INCLUDE, but are not limited to, fear, anxiety, anger, crying or, most importantly, a vagal reaction described above.

THE MA SHOULD REVIEW the specifications on the specific medication to be given. Are there recommendations on location, i.e. arms versus legs? What is the ideal depth of the injection, subcutaneous, subdermal or intramuscular? Injection depth pertains to how the medication enters the body. How fast should the medication be pushed? Is soreness or any other reaction to be expected? All these things should be determined well before the patient encounter.

HERE ARE the steps to perform an injection:

1. Assemble all the material necessary for the procedure.
2. Obtain consent from the patient.
3. Understand if your injection is subcutaneous, subdermal, or intramuscular.
4. Choose the site jointly with the patient, bearing in mind your experience of what is best tolerated or recommended. Patients often have a left or right preference. Be mindful of any special nerves or vessels nearby. Review anatomy with the doctor if necessary.

5. Fill the syringe with the medication as directed. Check for and dispel any air bubbles.
6. Clean the injection site with an alcohol swab.
7. Pinch the skin at the injection site to lift it.
8. Insert the needle into the lifted skin at a 90-degree angle.
9. Once the needle is in the tissue, draw back to confirm that the needle has not been inserted in a blood vessel. If, while withdrawing, you see a flash of blood into the syringe, remove the needle and choose another location. Bandage and apply pressure until bleeding has stopped.
10. Once a safe site away from vessels is confirmed, push the plunger to inject the medication. There is no need to rush.
11. Withdraw the needle and apply gentle pressure to the injection site with a clean cloth or bandage.
12. Dispose of the needle and syringe properly.
13. Observe the patient for five minutes.
14. Advise the patient to work the arm normally afterwards and even consider exercise involving the arm to minimize soreness.
15. Remind the patient that she may take acetaminophen and or ibuprofen.

IT'S important to follow proper hygiene and technique to minimize the risk of infection, side effects, and to ensure proper dosing. Office injections represent another convenience for the patient. Each office will have to weigh the pros and cons of offering them on site.

ORDERS AND SPECIMENS

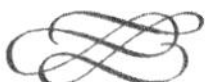

*O*rders and specimens fall largely within the purview of the medical assistant. Thus far, we have discussed the thinking based work that the medical assistant does. Now we are going to focus on something that is purely algorithmic, plug-and-chug, or cookbook, as we used to say in med school. Quality in preparing orders and specimens is essential; orders are commonly a matter of life or death. Getting the details 100% correct 100% of the time is critical. For this reason, we require looking things up over remembering, and checking and abiding by protocols over thinking.

MEDICATION ORDERS

While orders and specimens fall largely within the purview of the medical assistant, no medical assistant actually gives an order, officially speaking. Only caregivers such as physicians, certified nurse midwives and assorted other mid levels may do so. That said, it is routine for doctors to give verbal orders to medical assistants who then enter them into the system.

. . .

VERBAL ORDERS INTRODUCE a layer of convenience, but they also introduce potential for error. It is incumbent upon the doctor in question to verbalize herself clearly and precisely or else put her order message on a sticky note. It is still much faster for the doctor to put the medication, dose, and all the specifications on a sticky note than to fire up a slow computer, get on the right page of the right interface, and enter orders. Asking your medical assistant to enter orders may seem like a dump, and it most definitely is, but it is a dump that often keeps the clinic running on time. If the doctor has time and sees that the medical assistant is busy, it is common sense and common courtesy for her to enter the orders herself.

PRE-PRINTED order forms were a big step in the right direction to minimize errors in order writing. Computer interfaces for digital order entry have taken this a quantum leap further and are improving every year. These interfaces not only keep their selections to correct doses but also incorporate precautions and allergy crosschecking in their interfaces. The more sophisticated software also checks for medication interactions for a given patient.

ALL MEDICAL ASSISTANTS should briefly observe a moment of silence for all older physicians. This is because "in the olden days", we suffered through a great deal of pharmacology memorization that most of us probably forgot and that now is obsolete or automated. We had tiny reference books with miniscule print which we carried around. Perhaps we remembered more then because of the practice. Perhaps we forget more now because of the technology.

WHAT FORGETFUL PHYSICIANS do remember is that the devil is in the details. Exact doses matter. Exact dosing intervals matter. Medication interactions matter. We physicians also remember the names of all the medications that sound like one another and that are easily confused. We remember these, because they were always on the test. All of us, physicians and medical assistants alike, must respect the pharmacology.

MOST OF US carry cell phones and have apps. There should be no excuse for a physician or a medical assistant not to have a quick way to look up a medication. One of my favorite apps is Epocrates. It is worth calling your hospital's pharmacy to see what medication apps they recommend. On that note, there is nothing wrong with picking up your cell phone and calling your hospital pharmacist if you have a question. If you're not careful, you can learn a lot. The pharmacists appreciate our questions because it gives them confidence that we are trying to be careful and precise.

THIS BRINGS up the issue of medication errors. What if a medication order is found to contain an error? There is no office where it does not occasionally happen. Such an incident usually involves a lot of stress. Most such errors do not need to entail such high levels of angst. **We know and patients know no one is perfect.**

. . .

THE WAY TO avoid the angst is to report and disclose the error as soon as possible. This is the case whether the error was on behalf of a mid-level, such as a medical assistant or a physician. Basically, everyone needs to know about the error, from the caregivers to the patient and even, in some cases, the front office.

TRANSPARENCY IS GERMANE TO TRUST. **More importantly, it is critical to safety.** The patient needs to be notified as soon as possible so that she can stop taking the incorrect medication and begin taking the correct type or dosage. Any untoward effects of the error must be determined and watched for. If the error or the consequences of the error are serious, it should be reported to the office's Medical Malpractice Insurance carrier.

IMPORTANTLY, an apology should be issued from the highest ranking person in the office, either the office manager or the caregiver. No one person should be thrown under the bus, even if one person is responsible. An office functions as a team, and the team should bear responsibility. That said, the patient should be assured that a review is underway, as indeed there should be. An office record should be kept of any errors and their follow up. This should be confidential and for office use only.

APOLOGIES ARE NOT ONLY common courtesy, but they are associated with a higher degree of patient satisfaction and are inversely correlated with the risk of lawsuit.

· · ·

IMAGING AND CONSULTATION orders

ORDERS MAY ALSO BE for imaging or consultations. If orders for imaging or consultations are not made correctly to the consultant departments, the consult may not get done. While phone calls to consultant offices are time consuming, they are often illuminating and answer questions for many patients to come.

IMAGING ORDERS CAN BE VERY particular and must include things like right or left, with or without contrast. It is important for office staff to remember that staff at the consultant's office are there to help us use them correctly.

SOME FORMS of imaging require the patient to meet certain conditions. For example, gallbladder ultrasound requires a period of food abstinence beforehand. Pelvic ultrasound requires the patient's bladder to be full. Mammography is best done when there is no deodorant in the underarms. The medical assistant must possess all this knowledge.

REFERRALS

The trouble with ordering referral consultations is that the method is different for every office. This can even be true in a single university system. It is best to be familiar with the particular protocols at any office that is utilized. We in our OBGYN office commonly use many consultants from psychiatry, rheumatology, endocrinology, to physical therapy, general surgery, and everything in-between.

. . .

SOME OFFICES ARE "WALLED GARDENS". They make it very hard to get your patient in. These tend to be understaffed, overwhelmed offices. However, you are your patient's advocate. If your caregivers feel strongly about the necessity of the referral, you will do what it takes to get your patient into that office. This commonly requires a doctor to doctor conversation.

BEFORE YOU EVEN CALL THE office on behalf of your patient, let her know it is tough to get in and that she needs to be flexible with the times and days she will accept. This is called expectation setting and will help you on both fronts. Make sure your front office sends their front staff a thank-you note for their helpfulness. Consider bringing them a plate of holiday cookies every year

AS AN ASIDE, our office's thank you notes are preprinted. This makes it easier for staff to send one to anyone who has been helpful. People are not thanked enough and will notice. These cards have our distinctive logo and contain information about our practice, the types of patients we handle, and the types of surgeries I do. Thus, they also serve as an advertisement.

SOME CONSULTANT OFFICES want certain studies done and in the system before they see the patient. This ordering footwork falls to the referring office, i.e., the MA and her caregiver. This must be explained to the patient. The studies and the consultation all need to be arranged on a timeline that works for the patient. This too falls to the MA.

SPECIMEN HANDLING

Specimens are like orders in that the devil is in the details. The first order of business is getting the specimen packaged and labeled properly. Certain specimens need to go in certain collection media, such as a liquid in a tube. Every medical person in an office should be able to identify what tube is for what purpose. Laminated colored photographs with the tubes identified should be posted in all strategic locations. Despite this, specimen containers in drawers in each respective examination room should have their buckets labeled.

RECENTLY, at our center, a red top tube was for Group B strep. For reasons which are beyond my understanding, a red top is now for viruses such as herpes. No announcement was given; no reason was offered. The color was changed. You can't make this stuff up. This type of institutional error will happen. Watch for it. It's not very much fun for anyone to call a patient and say, "Please come back. We have to obtain that specimen all over again."

THE SPECIMEN CONTAINER should have a label. Some labels are stickers which you apply after the fact. Either way, all the requested labeling information should be supplied. Incorrectly labeled specimens are a big liability and a lot of work, because, after all, that result belongs to someone. What if it is abnormal? Who will you call? How will you follow up? All labelling irregularities have to be tracked down completely.

. . .

HANDLING laboratory specimens generated in the office also depends on your method of getting specimens to the lab. Some offices use the MA as a courier, and some labs send a courier as part of the service. Either way, the medical assistant has to have a sense of the timeliness and perishability of any laboratory specimens she may have to handle. For example, donor sperm used for artificial insemination is both time and temperature sensitive.

ANY DAY in a women's care clinic is bound to generate many specimens, all of which have to be handled promptly and correctly. Every medical assistant has to become an expert in specimen labeling, storage, and handling.

A PHILOSOPHY OF GIVING RESULTS

A seasoned MA will learn a great deal about her medical field. Yet will she know enough to speak for her doctor, her administrative team and the profession as a whole? No one should be expected to know all of this. Yet, that is what patients either consciously or unconsciously expect. The MA must bear this unreasonable expectation in mind. Her expertise is knowing how to recognize patient anxiety, declare her limitations in explaining results, and summarizing results without omitting or distorting key details.

PATIENTS HAVE concern or even anxiety about calling for their results. The whole idea of coming in to the doctor is anxiety producing. Patients come in to be scrutinized with tests and exams expressly to find something wrong. When it's time for the results to come in, anxiety is at its peak.

· · ·

With normal results, it is easy. The phone call for normal results can begin with the phrase "I have normal results for you." It could also start with, "Hello, I have good news." This puts people at ease. For results which are mixed but still not bad, one can say, "I have results for you… nothing bad, though." These phrases protect the patient's emotional state during the conversation.

For questionable or bad results, it is more challenging. Questionable results usually mean more studies will be necessary. When a patient enters the practice, she should be taught that medical care and medical testing is a stepwise process. Even an annual exam is a process because it involves more than the in-person visit. There are follow up screening labs and imaging, and the follow ups to those.

When all these things come back, there is usually something to talk about. If it is minor, it can be discussed over the phone. If it is anything but minor, both the patient and the doctor deserve an in person follow-up visit. From the patient's point of view, she gets the doctor's full attention on her and her issue. She gets the opportunity to ask questions in real time. From the doctor's point of view, she gets to confirm that the patient understands the results, their implications, and their follow up. She ends up with a better informed patient and less medicolegal risk.

For truly serious results, the doctor should deliver them. The MA should not be saddled with something of this nature. This is because the stakes are much higher for both the patient and the doctor. The consequences of giving the wrong impression or the wrong advice are higher.

WHEN A DEVASTATING DIAGNOSIS IS MADE, it is hard to imagine discussing it with the patient. The way to do it is to focus on the steps going forward. Naturally, the patient will be inclined to focus on the diagnosis, but her attention should be directed to the plan. Hope lies in the plan. The plan is action and action mitigates anxiety.

THE PLAN after any given sinister diagnosis usually involves new consultations with additional specialists, more labs and more imaging. It can go on to surgery. It is almost as though the patient needs a map or a timeline. The MA can help with this, even if the patient's plan is multidisciplinary.

IN THE SHORT-TERM, many patients, when given serious results either in person or on the phone, temporarily lose their ability to think or retain information. If, on a phone call, the caregiver senses this has occurred, she should try to arrange an in-person visit as soon as possible, bearing in mind the patient's distress. She should request that the patient brings a support person if possible, as well as pen and paper. This trusted second party can help clarify, take notes, and remember the details of the visit.

LIKEWISE, on such a visit, a doctor should have an MA present for the same purpose. In this circumstance, the MA is both a scribe and a chaperone for the doctor. We have all heard of doctors taking chaperones in with them to guard against allegations of physical or sexual impropriety. The chaperone also guards against allegations of communications impropriety, e.g. "I was never told…., You never said I had to…". If the patient does not have an appropriate support person to bring with her, the key points of her visit should be written for her. They should also be recorded in her chart. At the end of the visit, she should be given a copy of her visit note, either on paper, by email, or both.

OTHER RELEVANT MATERIALS may be given to the patient at the end of the visit. Examples of this might be a handout on the prevention of constipation, complete with personalized annotations about the patient's favorite foods for this purpose. While the handout need not go into the chart, a note that the handout was given must be made.

RESULTS AND CALLBACKS are a critical part of closing the loop. MAs and doctors must work together to achieve closure, which is intrinsic to high quality medical care, good outcomes, and defensibility against medical malpractice claims. With all results, the only acceptable method is to close the communication loop promptly and definitively. The policy that "no news is good news" is not a policy at all and should never be used with patient results, even if those results are normal. It is our policy to try to "empty the results bucket" every day. This is the case for normal and abnormal results.

GOOD OUTCOMES COME NOT ONLY AS BETTER medical treatments. They also manifest as more peace of mind for the patient. She is confident that her issues have been addressed. She comes away knowing she has been heard and evaluated, and that she has a plan.

GIVING OBSTETRICS RESULTS

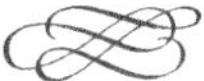

*P*renatal care is a process. It is scheduled, stepwise, and evidence-based. It comes from a synthesis of recommendations from bodies like the CDC (Centers for Disease Control) and the American College of Obstetricians and Gynecologists (ACOG). Certain things are done at prescribed times, be they ultrasounds, laboratory studies or vaginal swabs.

PATIENTS ARE BEST SERVED if they know what to expect at each visit, know how to follow through with the requested studies, and are notified of the results and implications of said studies. Medical Assistants play a key role in helping patients receive and remember their results.

TO GIVE a lab result or imaging report is easy. To put those test results properly into context is more challenging and more valuable. The obstetric patient will go through a series of planned tests at specific gestational ages. She will want and need to know the results of all of them.

FIRST TRIMESTER RESULTS

One of the first tasks in prenatal care is establishing dates. The MA takes the initial history of the last menstrual period as detailed above. The first trimester, which lasts until about 12-13 weeks, is the best time for establishing dates. Patients can still remember their period, and ultrasound is more accurate than later in pregnancy. Dating is usually established by comparing menstrual and ultrasound dates. Reporting this result sounds simple, but it takes some understanding of radiologic practices to explain it to patients.

AS DESCRIBED ABOVE, there are two pregnancy dating conventions. In academic embryology, embryologic dates are taken from the date of conception whenever that is in the cycle. The date of conception is not immediately apparent. In the medical field of obstetrics, dating is done from the first day of the last menstrual period (LMP). This is because the LMP is a knowable date.

FOR EXAMPLE, an embryo conceived on January 1st is literally 4 weeks old on the 28th of January. However, the obstetrician calls it a 6 week gestation since she dates if from the patient's last menstrual period which was December 19th, two weeks earlier than the conception.

WOMEN GENERALLY OVULATE (produce an egg) on day 14 of their cycle, where day one is the first day of their last period.

However, in some patients, the timing of ovulation can vary from about day ten to many weeks. This interval before ovulation is called the follicular phase, the time during which the follicle is ripening. The length of the follicular phase can vary widely.

THE PERIOD COMES fourteen days after the ovulation. This interval does not vary. The time after ovulation and before the period returns is called the luteal phase. It is always 14 days long.

A 28 DAY cycle implies an luteal phase of 14 days, an ovulation on day 14, and a follicular phase of 14 days. A 32 day menstrual interval implies a 14 day luteal phase as always, an 18 day follicular phase, and a day 18 ovulation. Because the luteal phase is always 14 days long, it is possible to count back fourteen days from the first day of the period to discern the day of ovulation of the preceding cycle. This is useful to determine the timing of ovulation in cycles of any length as long as they have consistent menstrual intervals.

THIS INSIGHT IS, however, retrospective. If a cycle is irregular, one cannot accurately infer the date of ovulation based on the prior pattern. This is where ultrasound becomes useful.

A TINY EMBRYO of less than 6 weeks gestation is difficult to measure for dates. However, it is at least possible to prove that the gestation is an intrauterine gestation rather than a tubal pregnancy. It is also possible to demonstrate heart tones, which reassures and delights the patient.

. . .

Shortly after six weeks, it is possible to make meaningful dating measurements. **Earlier ultrasound (US) is more accurate for dating than later ones.** In particular, first trimester ultrasound is accurate to within about a few days. Second trimester ultrasound is accurate to within one to two weeks. Third trimester ultrasound is accurate to within only about three weeks. Third trimester ultrasound is therefore not very useful for dating. It is only useful for growth trends, fluid measurement, fetal presentation, and certain other real time indicators of fetal well being.

Medical assistants will often note that patients are confused by late pregnancy ultrasound reports because they believe that their due date is actually changing. It is unfortunate, but understandable, that ultrasound reports speak of fetal size using weeks. For example, if the ultrasound techs report that a baby we know to be 30 weeks is measuring 35 weeks, it means the baby is actually measuring the size of an average 35 weeker. In other words, this baby is five weeks ahead in growth. Of course, this does not suddenly make him five weeks older. Medical assistants must be aware of this because sometimes patients get a little insistent that they are due earlier than they really are.

Prenatal care starts with the history of the menstrual period. Once that is established, an ultrasound can be ordered. Medical assistants fielding phone calls from newly pregnant patients need to have a rough idea of when to order a dating ultrasound and when to get the patient in for prenatal care. To do this, they need to take a good menstrual history.

IT IS stressful for everyone to inadvertently send a patient to ultrasound before the pregnancy can be visualized. A positive pregnancy test with an empty uterus on ultrasound raises concerns for miscarriage and ectopic pregnancy.

WITH A REGULAR PERIOD and a firm date of last menstrual period, dating can be approximated. An ultrasound at about 7-8 weeks can be scheduled. If there is reason to believe that the patient is farther along than that, an ultrasound should definitely be scheduled. If the patient's periods are irregular, a quantitative HCG level can be ordered. HCG is human chorionic gonadotropin, a hormone produced by the placenta. Once it gets to a level of about 1750 mIU/mL, the pregnancy should be able to be visualized on ultrasound and thus dated.

ESTABLISHING DATING criteria is one of the primary tasks of the first trimester. The second is accomplishing the prenatal labs. Prenatal labs consist of bloodwork and cervical swabs. These are usually performed during the first prenatal visit. It is usually possible to review the prenatal lab results at the second prenatal visit.

PRENATAL BLOOD WORK includes blood type and antibody status. Blood type is classified by the letters A, B, AB, or O. It also includes Rh status, which can be positive or negative. Rh status is of immediate importance. Fifteen percent of people are Rh negative. The rest are Rh positive.

IF AN RH negative mother carries an Rh positive baby, the immune system of the mother can attack red blood cells of the baby. An immunization called Rhogam is given to block this serious reaction.

MEDICAL ASSISTANTS SHOULD NOTE that Rhogam needs to be given within 72 hours of any episodes which may be an opportunity for blood mixing between the mother and the baby. These would include spotting, trauma, or invasive procedures, such as amniocentesis. Knowing the blood type as soon as possible in the pregnancy can be very important.

IF THE PATIENT is Rh negative, a complete explanation is in order. Medical assistants are key in starting this discussion with the patient. Knowing about the potential for an adverse reaction between mother and baby is a powerful motivation for the patient to promptly report any spotting that she may have.

A CONSIDERABLE NUMBER of prenatal lab tests are for infectious diseases: gonorrhea, chlamydia, HIV, Hepatitis B, Hepatitis C, Syphilis, and HPV via the pap. Patients are anxious to know the results of these particular tests. This is because there are interpersonal as well as medical conse-quences to these results.

· · ·

IF INFECTIOUS DISEASE studies are positive, treatments and consultations may be needed. The MA's job is to inform patients of results and plans, and to document such in the chart. Her job is to close the loop on all these results.

WHEN INFECTIOUS STUDIES ARE POSITIVE, patients want to know when and how they caught it. In many cases, this is not possible. Many of these organisms can be acquired and stay silent for prolonged periods of time, even years.

FIRST TRIMESTER SCREENING takes many forms. Its purpose is to screen for any abnormalities in the growing baby. The testing is often handled through a perinatologist's office. It usually includes both bloodwork and ultrasound. Results are usually given through the perinatology office. The MA's job is to ensure the patient's information is getting back and forth between offices and to the patient.

SECOND TRIMESTER RESULTS

The second trimester is between 12 and 23 weeks. It is a relatively quiet time of the pregnancy. All the preliminary labs and dating should be done. At about 20 weeks, all the baby's organs are formed. This allows visualization via detailed ultrasound. This information allows the identification of any moderate or large sized anatomic defects, or other features which may be of concern. A report of the ultrasound usually comes back to the obstetrician. The MA may see the ultrasound report first. Anything but normal results should be called immediately to the obstetrician's attention.

. . .

ABNORMAL FINDINGS on a 20 week ultrasound are often incomplete. Sometimes these findings are not seen again on later ultrasounds. Alternatively, a full understanding of the findings might not be reached until the baby is larger, when the next scan can be done. Abnormal findings on a 20 week ultrasound are always cause for a sit down discussion with the obstetrician and the perinatologist if one is available.

THIRD TRIMESTER RESULTS

The third trimester is the time for more intense scrutiny. Prenatal care visits for low risk patients are typically every four weeks, unless complications, questions or difficulties arise.

ALL PATIENTS SHOULD KNOW how far along they are in weeks. This helps them comply with their visit schedule. They should also know their active diagnoses, their medications and doses. Finally, they should know if they are high or low risk. The MA plays an important role in helping them clarify and remember those things.

THE 28 WEEK visit is an occasion for a few other particular tests. These include a cervical exam, blood testing, a test for gestational diabetes, and RhoGAM injection for the Rh negative patient. It also includes discussion of postpartum birth control or sterilization.

AT 28 WEEKS, the cervical exam is performed in the absence of any symptoms of labor. Once in a while, patients will change their cervix without knowing it. This is true for both first timers, "primips" and women who have already had deliveries," multips". Those having their first child who are "silently" dilating may have an incompetent cervix, which no one could have predicted. Those with prior deliveries may have incurred cervical damage at the preceding delivery which rendered their cervix incompetent.

BLOOD TESTING at 28 weeks comprises a repeat CBC, complete blood count, as well as blood type and screen. The blood type is already known and will not change, but the "screen" is an antibody screen. Antibodies can develop any time in the pregnancy.

WE ALL HAVE MANY ANTIBODIES, but the ones we refer to here are mother's antibodies against the fetal red cells. Having a baby grow inside a woman is an invitation to antibody formation. Normally, this does not occur, because in pregnancy we develop special blocking mechanisms to shield the baby. However, the system is not perfect.

THE ONE HOUR glucola is a 50 gram glucose load followed by a blood sugar test precisely one hour later. It is critical that the timing of the test be accurate. MAs who have reviewed the day's schedule beforehand should make note of whoever is coming in for a one hour glucola. If they have to, they can see the patient before the doctor and get the glucola done on time. If the blood sugar level is above the threshold, patients go on to further testing, usually a three-hour glucose tolerance test. This is done to separate the true positives from the false positives for gestational diabetes.

. . .

AT 28 WEEKS, Rhogam is given to any woman who is Rh negative. The exception is a woman who can identify the father of her baby who is also documented to be Rh negative. As mentioned above, Rhogam prevents a reaction between mother's immune system and the baby's red blood cells. It is given at 28 weeks on the assumption that we cannot always know when this type of immune reaction might take place. We know it is more likely to take place with trauma to the abdomen, or when the patient has bleeding in pregnancy. But it can also occur in the absence of any event or symptoms.

TWENTY-EIGHT WEEKS IS a good time to bring up postpartum birth control or sterilization. Basic options can be discussed. Any preliminary questions can be fielded. This sets the stage for more detailed conversations at a later time.

DURING THE THIRD TRIMESTER, growth or amniotic fluid volume abnormalities may appear. If these things are suspected, serial ultrasounds can be performed. Risk factors for poor fetal growth include everything from smoking and hypertension to poor placental quality. Risk factors for abnormally accelerated fetal growth include diabetes and obesity.

HIGH RISK PATIENTS should not be concerned about the safety of serial ultrasounds. Ultrasound uses sound waves to distinguish between tissues. There is no radiation involved, such as with an MRI, CAT scan, or plain film x-rays. Patients voicing concerns about multiple ultrasounds can be entirely reassured that there is no danger to them or the baby.

THE 35 WEEK visit is also special. At that time, a GBS (group B strep) swab is taken from the vaginal and rectal area. Group B strep is a common bacterium which colonizes about 20 to 25% of all women of reproductive age.

GROUP B STREP does not cause as many problems for mothers as it does for babies. If a newborn develops an infection with Group B strep, it can produce a pneumonia or even sepsis which can be life-threatening.

GROUP B STREP CAN ALSO, in a smaller percentage of cases, produce a postpartum infection in the mother. Fortunately, it is easy to reliably prevent all these complications with appropriate antibiotics during labor. Group B strep is generally sensitive to penicillin, clindamycin, Keflex, or vancomycin. Unless there is a penicillin allergy, we choose penicillin because it is the most effective. After that, we can choose one of the other antibiotics with the benefit of bacterial sensitivities ordered at the time of the initial swab.

HERE AGAIN, the medical assistant has to be alert to the situation. When the MA is rooming someone for the 35 week visit when the group B strep swab will be taken, she should remember to ask about the patient's allergies. If the patient is penicillin allergic, she knows to order both the group B strep PCR, which is a quick genetic test, but also group B Strep antibiotic sensitivities should it be identified in the patient's system. Asking for sensitivities will then alert the lab also to produce a culture which will actually grow the bacteria and subject it to different antibiotics such as Clindamycin, Keflex and Vancomycin. The unique sensitivities of that patient's bacteria will be determined in the lab. The report that is generated and sent back to the office will rank the other non-penicillin antibiotics in order of their effectiveness. Come labor, the clinician can choose the most appropriate antibiotic based on that patient's allergies and the unique sensitivity of her particular group B strep.

THE EARLIER THE antibiotic is started after labor or rupture of membranes, the better. Medical assistants will note that when taking triage calls, this and several other reasons make it especially important for them to ask about leaking or gushing of fluid. Pregnant women have a lot of discharge, which may be normal or even something as simple as a yeast infection. However, if there's any hint that membranes could be ruptured, it is necessary to send them straightaway to Labor And Delivery to rule out this important possibility.

SINCE GROUP B strep in pregnancy changes management so critically, the care team, including the medical assistant, should make certain that the GBS positive patient knows that she carries it. The patient should also know that this requires her to receive antibiotics in labor. This will help her understand she is not one who can linger at home with her early labor.

THIRTY-FIVE WEEKS IS the time of the TDAP and RSV vaccinations. TDAP stands for tetanus diphtheria and acellular pertussis. RSV stands for respiratory syncytial virus, a particular concern to newborns. These vaccinations cover disease entities for which immunity is not permanent.

THESE VACCINATIONS during late pregnancy protect mothers, but they are particularly meant to pass immunity to the baby. These days, there is so much vaccine reluctance that we introduce these vaccines as ones "for the baby". Without these vaccines, babies are born without immunity to these common but serious diseases. Passive immunity from mother's vaccine will last through the first two months of their life until they are old enough to get their own vaccinations. It is usually the responsibility of the MA to make sure that vaccines like these get done and documented in a timely fashion.

IN THE LAST four weeks of pregnancy, it is typical to perform a cervical exam at each visit. Therefore, in this time frame, medical assistants should know to have the patient undressed from the waist down. This is necessary to assess for cervical change but also to confirm that the baby is head down, also known as vertex presentation. The medical assistant will have asked all her typical questions about leaking, bleeding or decreased fetal movement. If the patient has had any hint of rupture of membranes, the cervical check is not done. Instead, in our center, she is sent directly to labor and delivery for a specialized test for rupture of membranes.

IT IS up to the medical assistant to have asked the key questions before the exam so that she can promptly report to the doctor any question of rupture of membranes. This is to prevent the doctor from going into the room and checking the cervix in the presence of early rupture of membranes. Ideally, the doctor queries the patient as well, since it is best to have two layers of safety. We avoid checking the cervix in the presence of rupture of membranes remote from labor. Doing so can increase the risk of infection during and after labor.

THE MA CAN PUT the patient at ease by reminding her about the routine cervical exams toward term. People dislike being surprised with examinations. It is better if they know what to expect. The results of the cervical exam should be reported and explained to the patient. She should be encouraged to remember it.

WHEN PATIENTS ARE near term or having discharge, they should be placed on a fluid proof barrier on the table. If the MA's initial intake history identifies these factors, the table should be dressed accordingly. Similarly, she should also provide pad liners for the patient to use when she dresses. This is because examination gel invariably adds to the discharge and can make a mess on people's clothing. These small conveniences enhance the patient's experience. They are squarely within the purview of the medical assistant.

BY THE TIME a patient comes in for her 36th or 37th visit, she should know her own group B Strep status. The MA can assist her by reminding her of this at each of her later appointments. The MA can also help remind the patient of her blood type, particularly if she is Rh negative. She can also help clarify the meaning of terminology, such as that used to describe the cervical exam. Patients late in pregnancy can have a tendency to go back-and-forth at odd hours to labor and delivery because they are concerned they might be in early labor. For them to have a clear concept of their last cervical exam will help other caregivers determine whether interval cervical change has occurred.

BY FULL TERM, a pregnant patient from a well run clinic should have a clear idea of herself as a patient. She should know her dating criteria, the results of all her prenatal labs, her blood type, her GBS status, her list of complications if any, her allergies, her meds, and her cervical exam. She should be able to recite the list of precautions requiring her to call in or go in. This would be an ideal patient indeed, and she would be so because of the persistent efforts of everyone in the office, especially the MA.

GIVING GYNECOLOGY RESULTS

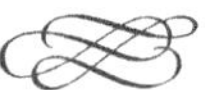

Gynecology results are just as important as obstetric results. Patients receiving gynecology results are just as anxious as those receiving obstetrics results. It is the job of a medical assistant to give that information as soon as possible. *Patient satisfaction depends on closing the loop in medical care.*

PATIENTS WANT to know the significance of all that was investigated during their visits. It is great to have an app that links directly to the healthcare system where patients can see their results. However, the real opportunity is for a knowledgeable person to communicate with the patient about their results.

MANY VISITS ENTAIL ORDERING numerous important tests. The return of these results is often enough to warrant a follow-up visit with the doctor. When this can be anticipated, a follow-up visit should be scheduled at the time of the original appointment. Less consequential results can be dispensed over the phone or by letter through a capable medical assistant.

GYNECOLOGY RESULTS FALL into the following categories: pregnancy tests, routine screening labs, and labs for specific conditions. Any problem oriented set of labs and imaging studies which will then lead to a course of action should be followed by a face-to-face follow-up visit with the doctor.

ROUTINE SCREENING TEST RESULTS IN GYNECOLOGY

Normal results from routine screening tests may be discussed over the phone.

ROUTINE LABS COMMONLY INCLUDE A CBC, the complete blood count. This includes the white count, which often pertains to infection, the hematocrit, which is the percentage of blood composed of red blood cells, and platelet count.

ROUTINE LABS also include the comprehensive metabolic profile or CMP for short. This includes the electrolytes such as sodium and potassium, blood sugar, kidney function tests, and liver function tests.

LIPIDS INCLUDE TOTAL CHOLESTEROL, which is then fractionated into high-density lipoprotein or HDL for short, the "good" kind, and low-density lipoprotein, or LDL for short, the "bad" kind. Included with the cholesterol subfractions is the triglyceride level. Both triglyceride and choles-terol levels pertain to heart disease risk. Triglyceride levels seem to be more predictive of heart disease in women than men.

ROUTINE LABORATORY STUDIES done at an annual examination also commonly include the TSH or thyroid stimulating hormone. This indirectly assesses the thyroid functioning. The thyroid gland governs metabolism.

MANY PRACTITIONERS in northern climates have added vitamin D to their routine laboratory studies. This is because vitamin D deficiency is endemic in these regions because of fewer hours of sunlight. When the MA calls the patient about her vitamin D deficiency, it is a good time to explain the importance of vitamin D.

VITAMIN D IS intrinsic to bone metabolism, but it also plays a role in immunity and perhaps mood. Patients may say that all they need to do is to get more sunlight. MAs can explain that the amount of sun needed to raise their vitamin D would be too much for their skin. While 20 minutes per day of sun is fine, the rest of the vitamin D requirement should be met through vitamin D rich foods like cold-water fish, lower fat dairy products and leafy greens high in vitamin D. *MAs should always be on the lookout for teaching moments and this is a prime example.*

STI SCREENING RESULTS

Any patient who has come to your office for prenatal care will have had sexually transmitted infection disease screening regardless of symptoms. However, it is recommended that asymptomatic non pregnant women in their twenties be offered chlamydia screening concurrent with pap, since chlamydia is so common in that population. Chlamydia screening is important for women because chlamydia is known for its tendency to produce scarring in the fallopian tubes, which can lead to pelvic pain and infertility. If the patient understands the offer of screening as a routine practice that is not particular to her, then she is more likely to be amenable to it.

GIVING results for STI screening requires sensitivity and forethought. Positive results may come as a surprise. The patient may feel it means her partner has cheated on her, which may or may not be true. Many STIs can go dormant for prolonged periods of time without symptoms. Some partners who pass STIs to new people do not know they carry it. The notification phone call should be in three steps. First, the patient should be allowed her reaction, within reason. Second, answerable questions should be answered. Third, treatment details should be discussed.

PAPS, COLPOSCOPY AND HPV DISEASE RESULTS

The Pap smear is so ingrained in the consciousness of the modern woman that it is sometimes confused with the entire annual check up examination itself. The Pap smear is actually only a single test, performed by brushing the surface of the cervix and the distal cervical canal with a small tool, which is then shaken into a liquid solution and sent to the laboratory. There, it is processed, literally "smeared"onto a slide, so that an automated system and a human cytotechnologist can review the appearance of the cells in the specimen. They are searching for pre-cancerous changes due to the activity of the human papilloma virus.

As IMPORTANT AS this and its results are, it remains a source of confusion. The pap looks at detached cells, cells detached by the brush that is used across the surface of the cervix. If the Pap shows any significant abnormalities, biopsies are performed. Biopsies, by contrast, are chunks of cells, however small.

SINCE THE PAP smear is easy to do and cheap to perform, it is an ideal screening test. However, as a screening test, it does not give definitive answers. Biopsies do. Therefore, after an abnormal Pap smear is reported, we ask patients to go to a procedure called colposcopy, as described in earlier chapters.

UNDERSTANDING THE PAP SMEAR, colposcopy and their significance for the patient requires understanding the HPV virus. HPV is a common DNA virus which has over 100 subtypes. It is ubiquitous in the population, meaning over 90% of the population has serological evidence that they have "seen" HPV. This does not mean that over 90% of people will get HPV related disease. Not at all. People have immune systems and they fight off viruses every day. Sometimes however viruses get the upper hand, and that is where the gynecologist comes in.

·   ·   ·

HPV COMES in subtypes ranging all the way from those that cause nothing, to those that cause genital warts, mild dysplasia and finally to those that cause cervical cancer. We believe that cervical cancer is a disease that develops in a stepwise fashion from mild, moderate, and severe changes, to the full-blown cancer picture. That is why periodic screening is so crucial.

WHETHER THIS TAKES place depends on the interplay between the immune system of the patient and the virulence of the particular subtype of the virus. For this reason, women are screened for high-risk subtypes of HPV. If they possess a high-risk virus subtype, the cytology of their specimen is interpreted with more caution, and the threshold for intervention is lower.

MAS GIVING Pap results which are abnormal will be met with a host of questions. Patients may ask outright if they have cancer. This is people's biggest worry. They seldom have the concept of screening firmly established in their mind. It is the responsibility of the caregivers to explain it. Patients need to be told that an initial abnormal test does not guarantee a bad diagnosis. It is usually just an indication for further investigation.

ONCE PATIENTS GRASP that HPV is a sexually transmitted virus, they will undoubtedly wonder who they caught it from. It often falls to the medical assistant to underscore that these viruses are long-standing in the body. This means that the patient could have acquired the virus at any time in her life. The patient wouldn't necessarily show up with an abnormal Pap until years or decades later. This makes the virus pretty much untraceable for all practical purposes.

HPV CAN GO DORMANT like this because it is a DNA virus. Most people are familiar with other common DNA viruses, though they may not realize it. HPV is part of a family of viruses which include the herpes virus, both the genital herpes type and the cold sore type, the chickenpox virus, and Epstein-Barr virus (EBV), which causes mononucleosis.

EVERYONE UNDERSTANDS these diseases come and go, sometimes depending on the immune status of the patient. Patients need to know that HPV is something that they share with their partner. They also need to know that men manifest HPV disease far less often than women, and for most intents and purposes, are just vectors of the virus.

IF THE PATIENT has had biopsies related to an abnormal Pap smear, the medical assistant can deliver results if they return normal. It is not uncommon for abnormal paps, even in the presence of HPV, to yield a normal biopsy. Then it is the MA's task to explain the notion of a false positive test. It is also important for the MA to emphasize that even though this year's biopsies are normal, the human papilloma virus is in the patient's system and may produce dysplasia in the future.

· · ·

We have collectively decided that a certain percentage of false positives is a fair price to pay for high sensitivity. We are most concerned about not missing anything.

IMAGING RESULTS

Gynecology care usually involves quite a bit of pelvic imaging, usually ultrasound. Ultrasound studies can be done either abdominally or transvaginally. Unless there is a distinct contraindication to use of a transvaginal probe, a transvaginal ultrasound should be obtained. It is important that the patient be informed in advance that this is planned. She should be informed of how it is done, and reassured that it is hygienic. Ideally, she should see the machine including the probe before the procedure.

In gynecology, ultrasound is used to look at everything in the pelvis, but some things image better than others. In the uterus, we can measure size in three directions. We can also see growths like fibroids. Fibroids are benign smooth muscle growths which are very common. Approximately one in four white women and one in three black women have them. We have a saying about fibroids: "They don't cause problems unless they do."

Fibroids come in three varieties: subserosal, which means under the surface, submucosal, which means under the inner lining, and intramural, which means within the wall of the uterus. Those that are subserosal are are the least likely to produce symptoms. Those in the muscle wall can produce cramps and pelvic pain. Finally, the ones under the endometrium can contribute to abnormal bleeding.

. . .

THE FIRST AND most important thing a patient will want to know about their ultrasound findings is whether the findings are benign. However, ultrasound cannot make tissue diagnoses. That said, in almost all cases, something that is definitively identified as a fibroid will be benign.

ULTRASOUND IS USED to determine characteristics of the endometrium. In particular, we measure the thickness of the endometrium and whether it is uniform. Any endometrial masses are of interest.

TO GET a detailed look at the lining of the uterus, we augment an ultrasound with an injection of sterile saline solution into the cavity of the uterus before scanning. This gives a much more detailed look at the lining of the uterus because it shows the silhouette of any endometrial findings. This procedure is called a saline infusion ultrasound (SIS) or a sonohysterogram.

PATIENTS SHOULD BE INFORMED in advance that SIS is a crampy but brief procedure, on the order of a few minutes. While it is not obligatory, the patient may premedicate with ibuprofen 600 mg a half hour prior to the procedure. Patients will need a pad afterwards because of the passage of the saline and some spotting.

ULTRASOUND IS ESPECIALLY useful for determining the characteristics of the ovaries. That is because the ovaries are a mixture of solid and fluid filled structures called follicles. This contrast shows up especially well on ultrasound. We can count follicles for determinations related to fertility. Ovarian masses and cysts can be scrutinized and measured. They can be thin walled, solid or septated. Physical features revealed on ultrasound go a long way in telling us whether an ovarian mass is of concern.

MOST WOMEN WILL HAVE a persistent ovarian cyst at some point in their life. Most are thin walled, fluid filled by products of the regular process of ovulation. These types of cysts tend to go away on their own if they are not too big. However, ovarian tumors, while not always malignant, are a big concern. Any ovary mass that is complex and growing, especially in older women, deserves attention and work up. It is not uncommon for this work up to lead to surgery.

ULTRASOUND IS LESS REVEALING when it comes to the fallopian tubes. That is, of course, unless they are diseased and thereby enlarged. Fallopian tubes can become enlarged due to a blockage. Such blockages can come from past infection with an organism like chlamydia, or any form of pelvic infection. Blockages in the tube can cause the tube to fill with fluid. Such a tube will be enlarged and visible on ultrasound. It may not otherwise cause problems.

LARGE TUBES like this can twist or rupture, causing pain. Tubes like this can also get infected and fill with pus. Patients present with pain and a feeling of being ill. Having a tubal abscess (TOA, for tuboovarian abscess) like this can lead to serious illness and even sepsis, which is a systemwide infection that is life-threatening.

FINALLY, a tube can contain a pregnancy. Even these, when they are early, can be difficult to visualize. Once they bleed or rupture, it is still difficult because the whole pelvis is filled with a combination of clotting and non-clotted blood and structures are scarcely distinguishable.

ULTRASOUND PLAYS a pivotal role in gynecology, just like it does in obstetrics. However, gynecology more often requires that we move forward to a CAT scan or MRI. This is often when malignancy is suspected. In these cases, we are not only looking at the pelvic organs but at the nearby lymph nodes.

GYNECOLOGY PATIENTS who present with any type of pelvic pain are candidates for imaging. Once the workup gets to the stage of imaging, it probably also includes lab work. While the patient will need guidance from the medical assistant, the doctor is almost uniformly involved in a workup of this complexity. The medical assistant should lean on her physician to help her know how to guide the patient through getting her imaging. When results return, she must notify the patient within the scope of her position, then schedule her follow up visit for a more definitive discussion with the provider.

THE MA MUST LEARN several ways to explain results. She must also know how to state the boundaries of her knowledge and the scope of her practice.

.   .   .

GIVING patients an overview of important results is an art. The medical assistant has to tell the patient enough to introduce the topic and justify the return visit with the physician. She must take care not to give in to patient pressures to interpret the findings and propose the plans, which have not yet been made.

PHONE TRIAGE

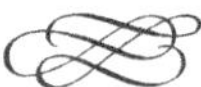

*T*riage is the process of performing a preliminary evaluation to determine the level of urgency.

PHONE TRIAGE IS BEST DONE in front of a chart, electronic or otherwise. The ability to reference the patient's history, photo, and lab results during a phone call is key. It is also good to have a pen and a notebook handy. Most medical offices now have an electronic medical record. Even so, I still favor the possession of a single spiral-bound notebook for taking notes during the triage call. The paper notes prepare the MA for the high quality note she will write in the EMR moments later, or the discussion she will have with her doctor.

IN A RELATED VEIN, I dislike sticky notes with questionable handwriting stuck all over someone's desk. This is a recipe for problems, if not disaster. Crucial messages about patient care can get lost or go to the wrong place.

. . .

I AM NOT OPPOSED to sticky notes if they are used correctly. However, somehow sticky notes give the user some sort of license to write illegibly or diagonally or around the back of the note in such a way that the reader might not notice. Sticky notes are intrinsically attracted to the floor. They bend on their own. They get lost.

NOTEBOOKS, on the other hand, don't get lost. They give the writer plenty of room to write a complete message, and they are hard to bend. Notes are even available in the order they are written. Pages can be meaningfully dated. I feel so strongly about this that I supply spiral notebooks for my entire office staff. I get them different colors and attractive designs so that writing in them is a pleasant experience.

TRIAGE of any kind should be done systematically. The first step is to invite the patient to say her piece. Then, gradually focus the conversation by asking specific questions. Always be sure to include the following: time the sign or symptom started, the time it finished, whether it is constant or variable, its character, the location, the intensity on a scale of 0 to 10, accompanying symptoms, and what they have tried to alleviate it. Although this sounds complicated, asking these questions soon becomes second nature.

OBSTETRICS PHONE TRIAGE

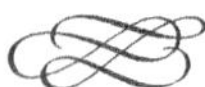

Obstetrics Triage

We joke and say that all doctors except OBGYNs are afraid of pregnant women. It's true. And they should be. This is because pregnant patients comprise two individuals: the mother and the baby. It is also because pregnancy takes most of the resources of the human body and throws them into one basket: the uterus. It and its contents becomes the largest, most vascular, and most dynamic organ that any physician or surgeon will ever try to manage. This is why OBGYNs need medical assistants.

FIRST TRIMESTER TRIAGE

First trimester triage includes the challenge of getting patients into prenatal care. Patients seem fairly willing to call once they have a positive pregnancy test at home, or if they think they are pregnant. Getting them into the clinic is sometimes another matter. Once people discover they are pregnant, they are eager to share it with someone, but not necessarily their whole family, or sometimes even the father of the baby. The office staff can be the first person they call.

THIS PHONE CALL to the office does not necessarily mean they are happy about the pregnancy. Medical assistants who field these calls should take a neutral tone until they understand the patient's feelings toward the pregnancy. Fully 50 percent of all pregnancies in the United States are unplanned. This does not necessarily mean these pregnancies are unwelcome. Even if a pregnancy is welcome, it still might be a shock. It is best to remain neutral until the patient sets the tone for the call. Possible examples of how to respond are:

"OK, how are you feeling? "

"OK, is this a surprise for you?"

"How are you adjusting to the news? "

"Do you know how far along you are?"

"OK, would you like to set up an appointment? "

ALTHOUGH THEY ARE CALLING, it is not always easy to get them into care. Obstacles to care include transportation and financial issues. Medical offices should have close ties with Social Work and related offices so that these challenges can be addressed early on.

DATING CONVENTIONS

It is worth reviewing that there are two dating conventions, embryologic dates which are done from the date of conception, and menstrual dates, which reference the first day of the last menstrual period (LMP).

As explained above, the clinical practice of obstetrics uses menstrual dates. Most women have something like 28 day intervals and generally ovulate on or near day 14. In this scenario, dates of conception are two weeks later than the LMP.

Patients often know when they conceived based on the timing of intercourse. Telling a patient her dates by this obstetrical convention may cause confusion and anxiety since she may not have had sex 2 weeks prior to her conception. The MA, armed with this detailed knowledge of dating conventions, can once again educate the patient and alleviate anxiety.

Since cycle length and timing of ovulation can vary widely in a minority of patients, calculations of pregnancy age must factor in variations in the length of the follicular phase. In confusing cases, ultrasound becomes the final arbiter of dates.

RULING OUT ECTOPIC

In our phone triage of first trimester patients, we are always concerned about the potential risk of miscarriage. However, we are far more concerned about the smaller but more dangerous risk of an ectopic, or tubal pregnancy. *While tubal pregnancies are more common when there are risk factors, anyone can have an ectopic pregnancy.*

RISK FACTORS for ectopic pregnancy are prior ectopic pregnancy, smoking, history of pelvic inflammatory disease (PID), history of chlamydia, or history of other intra-abdominal surgeries such as appendectomy, especially if the appendix was ruptured. These risk factors all share the common ability to create inflammation and scar tissue in the pelvis.

SCAR TISSUE in the pelvis or inside the tubes themselves is what predisposes the patient to ectopic pregnancy. The astute MA should always be on the lookout for signs or symptoms in the first trimester that could indicate the possibility of a tubal pregnancy. Ectopic pregnancy is a life-threatening condition that requires timely intervention.

THE SIGNS and symptoms of a tubal pregnancy can be difficult to recognize. They include, but are not limited to, pain, cramping, and any degree of bleeding. They can even be asymptomatic until the pregnancy gets relatively large compared to the pencil sized tube. I have seen an ectopic get as large as 12 weeks of gestation and have a heartbeat within the tube. This is a sad and very dangerous situation. Hopefully, the condition can be identified long before this stage.

· · ·

IF A PREGNANCY IS new and theoretically too small to be visualized by ultrasound, quantitative hCG (human chorionic gonadotropin) levels can be followed. In a normal pregnancy, these are expected to rise by about 1.75 fold every 48 hours. Quantitative hCG levels that do not rise according to this metric are suspicious not only for miscarriage but for ectopic pregnancy.

WHEREVER THE LOCATION of the pregnancy, a pregnancy should be able to be seen and localized on ultrasound if the quantitative HCG levels attain about 1750. Granted, it is harder to visualize a pregnancy outside of the uterus compared to within the uterus, but ultrasound, including transvaginal ultrasound, can usually do the job.

EARLY PREGNANCY TOXICITY TRIAGE

Once we are convinced that a pregnancy is located safely within the uterus, we can turn our attention to other concerns. Even if the patient cannot get into prenatal care as soon as we would like them, they can be counseled to begin avoidance of any toxic substances that they might normally encounter. These include but are not limited to occupational hazards such as chemicals or radiation, but also household items like volatile organic compounds (VOCs) in oil-based paints, pesticides or herbicides, or even the kitty litter box, which may contain toxoplasmosis, a parasite which is a known teratogen. Patients should be reminded to stay away from the most common toxins in our environment: tobacco, alcohol and drugs, including marijuana.

MARIJUANA IN PREGNANCY

The limited data available do not support an increased risk of congenital anomalies in women who smoke marijuana during pregnancy. Nonetheless, the American College of Obstetricians and Gynecologists (ACOG), the American Academy of Pediatrics (AAP), and the Academy of Breastfeeding Medicine advise avoiding marijuana use during pregnancy and lactation. This is because of concerns for the neurodevelopmental impact on the developing fetus and child. There is also data to suggest an increased risk of preterm birth and low birthweight. Cessation of marijuana use should be encouraged throughout the pregnancy. This type of counseling can start at the level of the MA and reinforced by everyone else on the team.

THE IMPORTANCE OF PRENATAL VITAMINS

Newly pregnant patients must be reminded to take prenatal vitamins which contain at least a 1000 micrograms (mcg), aka one milligram (mg) of folic acid. This is to prevent neural tube defects, a serious range of conditions involving the spinal cord and central nervous system.

UNHELPFULLY, prenatal vitamins are large and difficult to swallow. Many cause nausea. I have found that compliance is spotty with a traditional swallowed prenatal vitamin. For this reason, I've gone to recommending a prenatal vitamin in a gummy form. These are generally made with "natural" ingredients, include all the requisite nutrients, and are delicious. With this simple solution, compliance with prenatal vitamins is rarely an issue.

ACTIVITY IN PREGNANCY

Newly pregnant patients can still fall prey to the misconception that they have to stop exercising. This is false. ACOG has endorsed the continuation of exercise in pregnancy, barring specific complications such as preterm labor, bleeding, or high blood pressure. It is even advisable that a non-exercising newly pregnant patient begin mild-to-moderate exercise in pregnancy. Exercising consistently in pregnancy increases the likelihood of healthy weight gain, reduces the risk of gestational diabetes, and increases the likelihood of a normal labor and vaginal delivery.

Sports are a somewhat different story. Many sports can be continued in a mild-to-moderate form. With regard to equestrian pursuits, trail riding by an experienced rider on a well broke horse is reasonable. However, for the same patient, stadium jumping would not be advisable. Similarly, easy downhill skiing on groomed runs might be ok until halfway through the pregnancy, while bump skiing, aerials or racing would not.

Anyone can fall off their cross-country skis and twist an ankle. Anyone could fall and bump their head at the pool. The message is that all sports have some risk. Pregnancy introduces additional risk. ***If the sport involves large concussive forces that would come from impact or falls, then it is not suitable in pregnancy.*** Compromises to oxygen delivery, such as with high altitude sports and scuba diving are also inadvisable.

NAUSEA AND VOMITING IN PREGNANCY

Most early pregnancies entail some food aversion or nausea. Occasionally phone triage will reveal that a patient is not eating at all. Reports of not being able to eat or drink for a prolonged period should be taken seriously. Some patients will respond to oral medication, while others will need IV fluids at the hospital. The MA triaging such patients should determine if the patient is feverish, lightheaded or whether she also has diarrhea or has been able to make urine. The full report should then go to the doctor without delay.

PATIENTS SHOULD BE REMINDED to hydrate. Even those who cannot eat in the first trimester can often hydrate. MAs should remember that hydration is not limited to water. Patients can be encouraged to drink milk, kefir, herb tea, healthy smoothies, soup, soda water with natural flavor, and even Kombucha. In the same breath, MAs should counsel patients against consuming commercial sodas such as Coke, Pepsi, energy drinks, diet drinks, full sugar drinks, or otherwise.

SPOTTING IN EARLY PREGNANCY

Spotting in early pregnancy is serious until proven otherwise. It is a sign of possible impending miscarriage. At the same time, it is fairly common in normal pregnancies which eventually go to term. It can be associated with normal implantation. Counseling a patient who has called in to report spotting is a tricky matter. It is necessary to instill a sense of caution and a motivation to come in and get evaluated. However, it's also important to take a reassuring tone that is commensurate with the common and mostly benign nature of this symptom. Of course, light spotting is less concerning and more common than heavy spotting or heavy bleeding. While spotting is common, moderate to heavy bleeding in early pregnancy is not. While bleeding is common and happens along a continuum, heavy bleeding is worrisome.

ANY KIND of bleeding in pregnancy requires localization of the pregnancy. This means finding its location and thereby ruling out of a tubal pregnancy. As mentioned above, we draw serial quantitative hCG levels. If it is known that the pregnancy is far enough along to be visualized on ultrasound, an ultrasound is necessary. This is true even if an ultrasound was done for dating fairly close to the episode of spotting. Things can change quickly in early pregnancy and a determination of viability needs to be made.

SOME PATIENTS, and their family members, will resist coming in for spotting because they think nothing can be done. It is true that there is nothing we can do about an evolving potential miscarriage in the first trimester. However, patients and families need to be informed that miscarriage can come with complications for the mother, and that she needs to be monitored for her safety. There are many ways we can support and protect the mother during a threatened miscarriage.

WHEN SPOTTING IS REPORTED, it is critical to determine the Rh status of the patient. As mentioned above, the Rh status tells the clinician whether there is potential for an adverse reaction between the mom's immune system and the baby's blood cells. Spotting in pregnancy at any gestational age should be accompanied by a RhoGAM shot if the mom is Rh negative. This must occur within 72 hours of the spotting event in order to be effective.

PAIN IN EARLY PREGNANCY

Pain and cramps in pregnancy require investigation. Most people agree that early pregnancy produces symptoms of pelvic fullness and what some would describe as mild menstrual cramps. This is true even in the absence of spotting. Given that the pregnancy is a rapidly growing set of cells which essentially digs into the wall of the uterus to establish blood vessel connections, this makes sense. The pregnancy also sends out several different growth related hormones stimulating the uterus and its associated vasculature to grow and proliferate. While a few women have no sensations of early pregnancy, most people have the sensation of fullness, pressure or a little weight. Anything beyond that could be abnormal and should be investigated.

ANYONE in early pregnancy who has significant pain should be evaluated for an ectopic pregnancy. If an intrauterine pregnancy has already been demonstrated, the differential diagnosis still includes other concerning findings such as ovarian cyst or uterine fibroids.

A PREGNANCY always comes with an ovarian cyst. This is, of course, the corpus luteum. The corpus luteum is the empty egg sac where the egg for the pregnancy originated. After ovulation of the egg, the empty egg sac turns into a tiny gland-like body to secrete progesterone, which is necessary for the new pregnancy to survive.

MOST WOMEN DO NOT FEEL their corpus luteum. Sometimes, when the corpus luteum becomes excessively large or even hemorrhagic, it can produce pain. Corpus lutea are typically easy to visualize on ultrasound and can be readily tied to the source of the pain, reassuring everyone concerned.

OTHER OVARIAN CYSTS can arise in pregnancy. Not all of them are normal. There are specific criteria for evaluating the nature of any particular ovarian cyst. Ultrasound is the best initial way to assess these things. Ovarian cysts are common in pregnancy and they can produce pain. Even if large, most of them resolve on their own. With ultrasound, it is easy to follow them, and make sure there are no worrisome features. These worrisome features include mixed solid and fluid components, septations, irregular shape, or enlargement over time.

FIBROIDS CAN BE a source of pain in pregnancy. Fibroids arise more slowly than do most ovarian cysts. They are part of the uterine wall and can exist either on the inner lining, the middle of the wall, or the outer surface. Fibroids are relatively common even in young women. They are more of a nuisance than a threat in pregnancy. Large or particularly ill placed ones can predispose a patient to miscarriage or preterm labor, but the garden-variety small fibroids are usually well tolerated. That said, they can be uncomfortable as the pregnancy grows. Close monitoring clinically and through ultrasound are the approach to fibroids in pregnancy.

THE DIFFERENTIAL DIAGNOSIS of pain in pregnancy also includes urinary or bowel issues. Report of pain in a phone call to the office should prompt the MA to ask questions about these systems as well. In particular, the MA should ask about burning with urination, or any problems with bowel movements such as constipation or diarrhea. These symptoms get worked up just like they do outside of pregnancy.

PAIN IN PREGNANCY can also be musculoskeletal. The hormones of pregnancy, even early on, produce an increased laxity in the ligaments, which is adaptive to labor. This laxity produces an instability which, if not stabilized by strong musculature and good posture, leads to discomfort. The hips and low back region are particularly vulnerable to this kind of laxity related discomfort. Mechanical pain in pregnancy responds surprisingly well to regular physical therapy.

ONE OF THE most common types of mechanical pain in pregnancy is pain from the round ligaments. The pregnant uterus is like a hot-air balloon which is still tethered to the ground. It is filled progressively as the baby grows, gathering volume and causing a tightening of all the "ropes "which hold it down. In the front of the uterus, these "ropes" are the round ligaments. They tether the top "corners" of the uterus to the lower anterior abdominal wall in the right and left groin region.

. . .

WHEN THE UTERUS is small and not very heavy, it can't pull very hard on these ligaments. When the uterus is very large near term, the uterus has very little room to move. However, in the second trimester, the uterus is heavy enough to give a good tug and small enough to move freely. It is during the second trimester that MAs will take the most reports of pain in the right and left inguinal regions. Round ligament pain is sharp and can drop a patient to her knees. For this reason, it is also distressing. It can leave quite an ache for an entire week thereafter.

ROUND LIGAMENT PAIN IS MECHANICAL, in that it usually requires a movement to produce. Not uncommonly, a patient will report that she first experienced this pain as it awakened her from sleep. This is because rolling over quickly in bed can trigger it. Even though round ligament pain is fairly identifiable over the phone, caution should be exercised and the patient should be asked in for a visit at her soonest convenience if the pain is anything more than mild to moderate.

Round ligament pain is a diagnosis of exclusion. This means it is a diagnosis we can make after we have ruled out other more concerning possibilities. The differential diagnosis of round ligament pain includes early labor, urinary tract infection, adnexal mass, and kidney stones, to name a few.

CALLS ABOUT DISCHARGE IN PREGNANCY

Discharge in pregnancy can be symptomatic or asymptomatic. By this I mean discharge in pregnancy can simply be seen, or it can be seen and felt. Discharge that is accompanied by pain, itching or burning should always be evaluated by physical examination and laboratory studies if needed. Discharge that is suspicious for rupture of membranes should also be evaluated promptly. This is regardless of gestation. Rupture of membranes is not limited to late pregnancy. It can also occur in the preterm third trimester, or more devastatingly in the second trimester, but this is rare. Any watery, persistent discharge should be evaluated.

MOST PREGNANT WOMEN have more discharge in pregnancy. Normal discharge can range from mild to moderately increased in volume. Any copious discharge is probably abnormal. Discharge that is bloody is always suspicious and should be evaluated by physical examination in short order.

THE MOST COMMON forms of vaginitis that explain symptomatic discharge in pregnancy are yeast, bacterial vaginosis, and trichomonas. Yeast is bothersome, but the other two have serious perinatal implications. For this reason, we take reports of significant discharge seriously. MAs doing phone triage should note all the typical factors, such as characteristics of the discharge, including color, odor, consistency, sensations associated with it, and duration. This way the MA and the doctor can triage together to make sure that no concerning condition gets missed.

CONSTIPATION IN PREGNANCY

The medical assistant will field many calls about constipation, particularly from pregnant women. This is because constipation is common.

. . .

Constipation comes from suboptimal diet, sedentary lifestyle, and inadequate hydration. Add to this the pressure of the enlarging uterus and you have a real problem.

For the same set of reasons, constipation is relatively easy to solve. Modifications of diet, lifestyle and hydration are straightforward. However, diet, activity level and hydration practices are habits. **People have the habits they have for reasons.** These reasons are all the various constraints and patterns of their lives that have resulted in their present state. I won't say that changing habits is hard, but I will say it takes planning and perseverance.

Ideally, a patient with troublesome constipation should complete a food journal. Short of that, the medical assistant can ask about her last few meals and get a pretty good idea of her eating habits. From there, saturated fats and simple carbohydrates can be removed, and fiber, fruits, vegetables, and fluids can be added.

The same quick telephone assessment of activity levels can help guide recommendations. All pregnant women without complications should exercise regularly. The MA can review specific guidelines with them.

Finally, hydration can be quantified by using a large tumbler or thermos that are so popular these days. Failing that, the patient can simply titrate her water drinking so that her urine becomes clear and light colored.

. . .

ONCE NUTRITION, activity and hydration are optimized, few remain constipated. For those that do, there are fiber supplements and medications. There are laxatives, but those are to be avoided. Once patients are needing medication, the doctor should be consulted.

CONSTIPATION IS worth avoiding because it is uncomfortable. Moreover, it fosters the development of hemorrhoids which can be painful and require surgery. Such surgery can eventually damage the anal sphincter.

CONSTIPATION ALSO PREDISPOSES patients to urinary tract infections. It does so by pressing on the urethra and bladder, and preventing efficient bladder emptying. Urinary tract infections in pregnancy can lead to kidney infections, which can cause preterm labor.

ANSWERING THE UNANSWERABLE

Patients can have many pressing questions which they pose over the phone before their first prenatal visit or shortly thereafter. These cannot all be anticipated. It is never wrong for the medical assistant to bring these questions to the doctor. It is not uncommon for patients to ask questions that are difficult to answer or even questions that are unanswerable. The medical assistant needs to have a script in her mind about how to respond to tough questions. Having this script will help her respond to these inquiries quickly, effectively, and with less stress. For example, "That's a great question, but not one that I often hear. I will have to speak to the doctor about this. She may even have to do a little research to get you an answer. We will have to get back to you in a few days or you can discuss it at your next appointment."

IT IS NOT wrong to say, "I don't know". However, it is wrong to leave a patient hanging without knowing where to turn. The better way is to say "I don't know. But I will help you find an answer, if there is an answer."

SECOND TRIMESTER TRIAGE

When the patient reaches the second trimester, her prenatal care is well underway. Most of the preliminary studies, including bloodwork and imaging, are finished. The patient can relax into the pregnancy. Adverse outcomes are few in the second trimester. That said, when distinct symptoms are noted in the second trimester, they can be more serious.

PAIN in the second trimester can be from mechanical reasons, such as a strain on the round ligament as mentioned above. It can also be from persistent or new ovarian cysts or masses, but these are rarer.

PAIN in the second trimester can come from labor. We don't normally think of labor in the second trimester. This is because progressive uterine contractions strong enough to expel the pregnancy rarely come in the second trimester. When they do, they are usually the result of an undiagnosed incompetent cervix and or rupture of membranes. These are very serious conditions which have meaningful interventions. It is far better to bring a patient in to be checked than to brush off concerning or persistent symptoms. So much of this important triage falls to the medical assistant, so it is worth mentioning.

WE THINK of an incompetent cervix as being produced by a cervical cone biopsy or LEEP (loop electrical excision) done prior to the pregnancy. It would be a mistake, however, to think of patients with a history of LEEP or cone as the only ones who can have an incompetent cervix. Sometimes a congenital uterine anomaly is the culprit.

SOMETIMES PATIENTS GO until their first pregnancy before they realize that they have a uterine anomaly. A uterine anomaly can take many forms, from a heart-shaped uterus to one uterus with two horns, and finally an entirely duplicated system with two smaller uteruses side-by-side. There can be one normal cervix, two normal cervices, one incompetent cervix, or two incompetent cervices. There is no way for a first timer to know whether she has this type of anatomy unless it was evident on her physical examination. A first timer calling in with unusual pressure, discharge or crampiness in the second trimester should be brought in and examined. Most of these patients will be OK, or have something simple like a urinary tract infection. Some will merit extensive intervention.

PAIN from non-gynecologic or non-obstetric reasons is also an important consideration in the second trimester.

KIDNEY STONES SEEM to have a way of appearing in the second trimester. There seems to be some combination of poor hydration status and compression of the ureters which seem to make this diagnosis more than rare. Kidney stones present with pain that is in the flank, meaning the front and back of the sides, sometimes radiating and coming in nauseating waves. The urine may or may not be discolored or bloody. Patients characteristically state that they cannot get comfortable.

KIDNEY STONE PAIN, also known as ureteral colic, is miserable. Moreover, a kidney stone left in place in the ureter over time can damage the kidney. For these reasons, one never wants to miss the diagnosis of kidney stones. Other conditions, like appendicitis or ectopic pregnancy, can mimic kidney stone pain. These can kill you within the hour. Everyone in the medical office, including the medical assistants, needs to be aware of it.

,

Appendicitis comes in pregnancy just like it does outside of pregnancy. However, the pain from appendicitis may be a little higher and a little more decentralized in the presence of the pregnant uterus. Never think that because someone's pain isn't strictly in the right lower quadrant, that it can't be appendicitis. Typical appendicitis symptoms are pain as described, unwillingness to eat, nausea, vomiting and possibly fever or feverishness.

MEDICAL ASSISTANTS but also doctors and nurses of all stripes should note that when taking a history, feverishness, chills, and fevers, all count for the same thing. Any of this adds to the index of suspicion for appendicitis or other serious process. If there is a delay in diagnosis, an appendix may rupture. This produces a vicious peritonitis and can quickly lead to sepsis. Sepsis is a systemwide infection that affects the whole body. It is life-threatening and can lead to septic shock.

THIRD TRIMESTER TRIAGE

The third trimester is when most complications occur. Once again, phone triage is best done with the chart open and notebook in hand. If possible, the MA should review the patient's history prior to taking the call. Those who have had prior instances of preterm labor, preterm premature rupture of membranes, abruption or preeclampsia are at higher risk to repeat the same thing in subsequent pregnancies. That said, there is always a first time for everything, and even first timers need to be watched for these problems, particularly if they are very young, very old, or otherwise have risk factors.

TRIAGE FOR PRETERM LABOR

Medical Assistants doing phone triage for third trimester patients should understand that the presentation of preterm labor can be subtle and variable. Patients in preterm labor can report contractions, pressure, low back pain, diarrhea, constipation, or even just a general sense that something is not right. Preterm labor can come out of the blue but it can also be brought on by trauma, stress, infection such as urinary tract infection, or unappreciated rupture of membranes.

IN THE THIRD TRIMESTER, the possibility of preterm labor should be evaluated on labor and delivery. This is because its evaluation requires more than what is available in the office.

In particular, the assessment for preterm labor involves cervical exams to be done over a period of time, such as two hours. It also involves the ability to monitor for contractions.

TRIAGE FOR PREECLAMPSIA

The presentation of third trimester preeclampsia can be subtle. Preeclampsia is common, so it has to be watched for all the time. It is part of the spectrum of hypertensive disorders of pregnancy. This includes pregnancy induced hypertension, preeclampsia, severe preeclampsia, HELLP syndrome, and eclampsia. Another name for preeclampsia is toxemia. This spectrum of disease is always evaluated at Labor And Delivery.

THE SIGNS and symptoms of hypertensive disorders of pregnancy include, but are not limited to, headache, blurry vision, spots or flashes before the eyes, swelling in the face or extremities and right upper quadrant pain. Of all these, headache and extremity swelling are the most non-specific. Until the patient's normal pattern of symptoms is established, even these common symptoms need to be evaluated.

PREECLAMPSIA IS an inflammatory and immune based reaction to the pregnancy which affects the entire body. It can affect any organ, some more than others. It does damage at the level of the capillaries, the smallest vessels in the vascular tree. The kidneys, the brain and the placenta have a fine bed of capillaries which are vulnerable in preeclampsia.

. . .

BECAUSE PREECLAMPSIA AFFECTS THE PLACENTA, it affects the baby. It can compromise the blood flow and oxygen delivery to the baby. We can detect poor fetal oxygenation by looking at the fetal monitor strip on Labor And Delivery.

PATIENTS SENT to Labor and Delivery for "rule out preeclampsia" can expect bloodwork and a urinalysis. Bloodwork and urinalysis are done because preeclampsia has important short-term effects on the components of blood, and the markers of kidney and liver function. Patients also get serial blood pressures, since elevated blood pressure is the most common sign of nascent preeclampsia. All this can take somewhere between two and four hours. Patients should be informed of this so they can plan.

TRIAGE FOR RUPTURE OF MEMBRANES

Phone triage for rupture of membranes is not as easy as it would seem. Sometimes rupture of membranes presents as a slow, barely discernible trickle. Other times it is a big unmistakable gush of fluid. Normal amniotic fluid should look about like champagne. It should not smell like urine. Sometimes, however, it has a tinge of blood to it, especially at full-term. Sometimes, it has a greenish tinge, which indicates meconium.

MECONIUM IS the bowel movement of the baby. Near the due date, meconium is fairly common and not necessarily a reason for concern. However, any woman at any gestational age with any sign of rupture of membranes, whatever the color, should be advised to go to labor and delivery for prompt evaluation.

TRIAGE FOR GENERAL ILLNESS

Ordinary illness can intervene in the third trimester just as it can in any part of the pregnancy. The threshold for intervention is lower during pregnancy, even for the common cold or stomach upset. In these days of Covid, we spend a lot of time getting patients screened for that. Even if they screen negative for COVID, we still take their garden-variety illnesses seriously. Entrenched upper respiratory infection, particularly in pregnant patients who smoke or who are asthmatic, should be evaluated.

INFLUENZA A and B are especially dangerous in pregnancy, much more so than in young non-pregnant women. At the beginning, influenza looks like any other upper respiratory infection. Medical assistants doing phone triage should take note. Patients who are negative for Covid and negative for influenza should, once recovered, be vaccinated for both if they have not already been.

ANY KIND of gastroenteritis which is more than short-lived or suspicious for producing dehydration should be evaluated in a setting where IV fluids could be given.

TRIAGE TO ENSURE COMPLETE PRENATAL CARE

Patients routinely miss appointments and diagnostic studies. It often falls to the medical assistant to be alert to this. She can work with the front office to reach out to these patients to bring them back into the schedule in a timely fashion.

· · ·

JUST BECAUSE A PATIENT shows up to her appointments does not necessarily mean she has completed the studies that were ordered. The medical assistant is responsible for confirming that everything that was ordered got done and the results loaded into the prenatal record.

TRIAGE FOR THIRD TRIMESTER BLEEDING

Bleeding at full-term can be normal, but in this situation, a patient is guilty until proven innocent. All bleeding requires an evaluation. At full-term, it can be as benign as the "bloody show". This generally takes the appearance of "snot" with streaks of blood. If the patient is dilated, had recent intercourse, or was recently given a cervical exam, it is probably benign. However, such things have to be vetted with the physician. The evaluation of third trimester bleeding requires a visit to labor and delivery for a fetal monitor strip (NST, or non-stress test) as well as an additional cervical examination. The medical assistant has a critical role in reinforcing this logic, which, by the time of 40 weeks, should become second nature to the patient.

TRIAGE FOR DECREASED FETAL MOVEMENT

Decreased fetal movement also requires an evaluation. There are several ways to think about assessing this. First, it is important to acknowledge any pattern of fetal movement that deviates from the particular baby's norm. You can be sure that by the last month of pregnancy, the patient knows the baby's pattern. That said, there is a certain natural decrease in fetal movement after 37 weeks simply because there isn't very much space left to move. The ratio of water volume to baby volume gets smaller. Even considering this, all babies should have regular movements, however small, especially after meals. Any questions should prompt the ordering of a non-stress test.

IF A PATIENT HAS NEVER HAD a non-stress test, it should be explained in advance. Patients might be happy to learn that it is a restful procedure wherein they are required to lie in a bed with two belts on their belly, one to monitor the contraction pattern if it is present, and another to monitor the baby's heart rate. They are encouraged to eat and drink as they see fit. If the strip immediately meets criteria, the non-stress test or NST for short, it can take as little as 20 minutes, but it often takes closer to 40 minutes.

LABOR AND DELIVERY units vary in whether they take non-stress test patients on a walk in basis or by loosely scheduled appointments. NSTs for decreased fetal movement, bleeding, or rule out ruptured membranes are not elective and must happen promptly whether they are scheduled.

TRIAGE FOR TERM LABOR

MAs can also field questions about the beginning of labor. First timers (Primiparous patients or "Primips") obviously have the most questions. We tell patients that if they have contractions that take their breath away every 3 to 5 minutes for a solid hour, that they should be evaluated. We also tell patients that if they have any contractions of any duration or strength which are severe or accompanied by a strong and compelling downward pressure, that they should be evaluated.

. . .

MEDICAL ASSISTANTS CAN DO everybody a favor by finding out how far the full-term patients live from the hospital. This way, patients who are uncertain about the beginning of labor or who have a history of rapid labor can plan more effectively about their particular threshold for calling in or coming in.

THIRD TRIMESTER TRIAGE CONCLUSION

Obstetrics triage becomes increasingly complex as the pregnancy progresses. Often, the diagnosis takes more than one test and more than a little time. Doing obstetric triage and answering obstetrics questions is more of a process than one phone call. Educating patients early about this reality brings the patient onto the obstetric team.

THIRD TRIMESTER PHONE triage is a high-stakes business. Medical assistants should have a low threshold for checking with their physician right away when these calls come in.

GYNECOLOGY PHONE TRIAGE

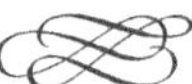

When a non-pregnant patient calls the office, we do not know whether her complaint will fall within the realm of gynecology. Her complaints might stem from pregnancy, among many other things. An open mind and the ability to question the patient skillfully are needed for safe phone triage.

WHEN TAKING A TRIAGE PHONE CALL, you are essentially taking a history. Classically, we are trained to ask open-ended questions at the beginning of the conversation, and then follow up with more specific questions later on. The old TV doctor's way was to begin with, "What seems to be the problem?". Nowadays, we are more likely to say, "How are you doing?", or, "What's going on?". The patient should respond with a complete narrative of what she has been observing. If she is hesitant, she should be encouraged to elaborate in her own way.

. . .

PATIENTS WHO FEEL REALLY POORLY MAY NOT articulate well. When a patient feels that badly, a family member or friend should bring them in for direct evaluation, either to the office, urgent care facility or the Emergency Room, as acuity dictates.

MANY PATIENTS WILL CALL in and say something completely non-specific, such as "I just don't feel good." It is tempting to dismiss these patients. However, it is very important to investigate further. A good way to focus the history is to ask about systemic symptoms. These are symptoms that affect the whole body. They would include fever, chills, and body aches, which are also called myalgias. After inquiring about systemic symptoms, one can ask about specific disease categories such as upper respiratory, urinary tract, or gastrointestinal issues. Most patients will be able to provide some guidance on what they are feeling and observing.

THIS LEADS me to a subtle distinction in nomenclature. A symptom is something that you feel, and a sign is something that you observe. For example, abdominal pain is something that you feel, whereas bloody diarrhea is something that you observe. Therefore, abdominal pain is a symptom and bloody diarrhea is a sign.

GYNECOLOGY PHONE TRIAGE may be hampered by social norms or interpersonal factors. Encourage the patient to be frank and clear about her symptoms and signs. If she is sounding unduly vague, it may be because she does not have privacy on the other end. If you sense this is the case, either invite her in to clinic or give her a chance to call back.

REFINING THE TRIAGE HISTORY

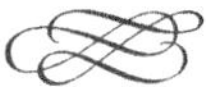

*R*egardless of the category of the illness, several increasingly specific questions can be asked. I ask about time first. It is important to know when the symptom started and what else was going on at the time. I also ask what percentage of the time the symptom is present and how long it lasts. Regarding a symptoms' severity, I like to know how mild it is at its mildest, how bad it is at its worst, and what it is on average. I like to do this on a scale of 0 to 10 with zero being none and 10 being the worst pain that the patient can imagine.

IT'S SOMETIMES useful to ask about the character of the pain, though this is not as useful as you might imagine. Particularly in the abdomen and pelvis, pain is poorly local-ized. This means that the actual source of the pain might be on the left but the patient experiences pain on the right, and vice versa. It can be informative for the patient to describe the character of the pain, in terms of whether it is dull or sharp, or both. Sometimes pain radiates. It is useful to know how the patient perceives this.

We like to know what modifies pain, i. e. what makes it better and what makes it worse. Classic questions would be, "Is it better or worse with any of these: eating, drinking, a full bladder, bowel movements, moving a certain way, breathing in deeply…?". Finally, we also like to know what the patient has done about the symptoms and signs thus far, and whether those measures have made any difference. I once had a professor who told me, only somewhat metaphorically, "If you listen long enough, the patient will tell you the diagnosis." She also said, "History is 90% of the diagnosis."

TRIAGE OF PELVIC PAIN

All of this history taking logic applies very well to pelvic pain. Pelvic pain, regardless of the source, can start out as dull or sharp. As it worsens, patients can localize it. As time passes, they learn more about its modifiers. Pelvic pain can be caused by such a wide variety of things that it simply requires an in-person exam.

TRIAGE OF VAGINAL SYMPTOMS

We get calls every day about vaginal complaints. This could be pain, itching, discharge, or odor. As tempting as it is to think that you know what's going on over the phone, it's best to have the patient come in for an examination and confirmatory testing. The most common vaginoses are yeast, bacterial vaginosis and trichomonas. They are not always easy to distinguish without specialized lab tests. The consequences of guessing it to be one and having it be another are multiple. The patient experiences extra days of discomfort and frustration. Expensive medication is wasted on the wrong diagnosis. The wrong medicine can even make the patient's condition worse.

ALL THIS SAID, there will always be the world traveling patient who is just about to get on a plane to go to Timbuktu, who just took a course of antibiotics for her tooth and now feels quite certain that she has a yeast infection. There is simply no way she can come in to be checked. In this case, the MA has to report the details to the caregiver in a timely fashion. She and the patient have to have a conversation about the consequences of guessing incorrectly, missing the diagnosis, and giving the wrong medication. If the patient is willing to take that risk and feels most comfortable simply picking up a prescription, then under these types of very constrained circumstances, administering a prescription over the phone can be acceptable. All the same, it is not ideal. We have noticed that it is the same patients repeatedly who paint themselves into these corners. At some point, the corner painting needs to be discussed.

TRIAGE OF URINARY SYMPTOMS

Pain with urination is a very common reason for calls to our office. Here, a full visit is not actually necessary. However, it is very useful to have the patient simply stop by to give a specimen. Most of the time, a well done clean catch urine specimen is all that is needed to confirm the diagnosis. Such a specimen can be dipped in the office then sent to the lab for culture and antibiotic sensitivities.

· · ·

WHEN THE PATIENT comes in to give her specimen, we remind her to drink enough fluid and void after intercourse. Relative dehydration and failure to void after intercourse are two of the most common reasons that we have seen for common urinary tract infections (UTI). We also ask about constipation, recalling that it is risk factor for UTI.

IN CERTAIN PATIENTS, clean catch specimens are inadequate. This would include obese patients. Similarly, pregnant patients often have a hard time with the clean catch technique. One special group is those patients who have recurrent urinary tract infections. In this population, a catheterization specimen is much more useful. In this group, it is very important to identify the specific bacteria that is causing the recurrent infections. Antibiotic resistance may have developed, and this must be ascertained in order to choose the correct medication. If the patient truly has recurrent urinary tract infections, the patient should see an urologist to identify any treatable underlying cause. In our clinic, it is like baseball. After three urinary tract infection "strikes" in one year, you're out…. to the urologist's office.

TRIAGE OF PAINFUL INTERCOURSE

We get a fair number of calls pertaining to pain during intercourse. Pain during intercourse is also called dyspareunia. This is a category which many patients are reluctant to discuss. If a patient has mustered up the courage to call about painful intercourse, it is probably significant pain and must be taken seriously and with sensitivity.

.   .   .

PAIN WITH INTERCOURSE is worse than pain elsewhere. It has emotional and social components. Care must be taken from the outset of the phone call to reassure patients that this is a common problem and that its evaluation is routine. The MA must always keep in mind the possibility of abuse. She should consult with her provider about how and when to ask about it.

EVALUATION of painful intercourse comprises all the history taking pertinent to urinary tract infections, vaginitis, pelvic pain and abdominal pain, all put together. It really exercises all the medical assistant's history taking powers. And yet the patient needs to come in. The patient must expect a pelvic exam, labs, and possibly imaging.

TRIAGE OF ABNORMAL PERIODS

Patients call in when their period has gone awry. Medical Assistants must have a basic understanding of what is normal menstruation. We may think what we have personally experienced is normal, but it is not necessarily so. The normal duration of menstrual flow is typically 3 to 7 days, usually five. The normal menstrual interval is defined as day one of one period until day one of the next period. A normal interval is 21 to 25 days with a mean of 28. Normal menstrual flow is defined as blood loss no greater than 80 mL per period. This volume is obviously difficult to ascertain. In practical terms, we ask patients if they have to change their super pad or tampon more than every couple of hours. If so, we consider that heavy. We have also found it useful to ask if the period is much heavier than it used to be. Interval change is an important clue.

. . .

MEDICAL HISTORY TAKING for abnormal bleeding must always include whether contraception is being used. If contraception is in use, it is important for the history to include the type. It is also key to understand where the patient is in the contraceptive cycle. With a birth control pill pack, it is important to know what pill the patient is on. For example, the patient can look at her pack and tell quickly that she is on the second pill of the third week. This helps the caregiver determine what could be wrong. Of course, patients with abnormal bleeding must be asked if any pills were missed. Even one missed pill can cause unscheduled bleeding.

ABNORMAL UTERINE BLEEDING after the first period and before the conclusion of menopause raises the possibility of pregnancy. This is the case even if a vasectomy or tubal ligation was performed. All abnormal uterine bleeding requires a visit in the office. However, even if the office cannot get the patient in that same day, it is prudent to rule out pregnancy by having the patient do a pregnancy test.

WHILE MOST OF the work up happens within the walls of the clinic, the laboratory, and the department of radiology, the initial phone call about abnormal uterine bleeding is important. Some bleeding is catastrophic. Certain patients will wait until their symptoms and signs are extreme before calling in. If there is heavy free flow, lightheadedness, or significant pain, she should be brought in by family or friends without delay.

PATIENTS WHO PREFER to wait until they are nearly dying to call a doctor are called, "under-reporters". Patients who call frequently about trivial things are called "over-reporters". Both are important patient behaviors which can lead to harm. It behooves the medical assistant and everyone in the office to be aware of these patient tendencies. Both under and over reporters respond well to education and face-to-face contact. At no time should any patient's concern be trivialized, even if they tend to "call wolf".

THE DIFFERENTIAL DIAGNOSIS for abnormal uterine bleeding is very large, too large to begin discussing over the phone. Once again, medical assistants will need to put boundaries on their conversations to discourage fruitless speculation, anxiety and wasted time.

AMONG OTHER PHONE call mysteries are lumps, bumps, and spots on the perineum. Because of privacy concerns and potential for inaccuracy, offices should not accept texts or email photos of these. Patients should be discouraged from showing us these during telemedicine visits. These entities have all the variety of human anatomy and pathology. They always require an in office examination and commonly require biopsy or consultation. Patients should be brought in for these without delay.

THE NUMBER of concerns about which patients call is limitless. There will come a stage when you think you've heard it all. Believe me, you have not heard it all and you never will. There will always be something new, something that will need to be figured out.

GENERAL MEDICAL TRIAGE

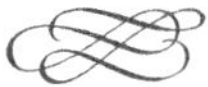

Obstetricians and gynecologists serve as primary care providers for many women. For this reason, patients call the office with complaints that do not fall within the realm of obstetrics or gynecology.

MOST OF THE TIME, they understand that we as OBGYNs do not directly take care of these problems. They simply recognize us as fully credentialed physicians and want our input on how best to proceed. In this manner, we provide a critical gatekeeper function for our patients. We can provide very effective triage. Because of our connections in the medical community, we can help make the best patient care plans even for conditions which are outside of our specialty. Medical assistants and others answering the phone should know how to field these calls.

COVID TRIAGE

This edition is written during the COVID-19 pandemic. COVID-19 promises to be an issue in the medical community for the foreseeable future. For this reason, we will discuss the pandemic awareness that must be brought to every triage phone call.

COVID-19 IS PRIMARILY A RESPIRATORY VIRUS. One expects that the primary symptoms would be respiratory. For example, this would mean a runny nose, sinus congestion, sore throat, cough, and the associated fevers and chills. However, a wide variety of symptoms can be attributed to COVID, including GI symptoms such as nausea, vomiting and diarrhea. Some COVID patients present only with loss of taste or smell. In any of these cases, the first step should be a test for COVID.

ANY MEDICAL ASSISTANT in any medical office during the pandemic should have a full understanding of all the sites nearby where COVID testing can be obtained. For each site which a patient may choose, she should know the details, such as whether appointments are necessary, or where to park. She should be able to give directions to each testing site. The medical assistant should also know how these results will reach the patient and the office.

THE COVID-19 PANDEMIC has brought another level of awareness of the spectrum of disease which viruses may cause. One of the most important and yet underemphasized effects of COVID-19 infection is hypercoagulability. This means that in the normal balance of our bloodstream, COVID-19 infection tips us pathologically toward abnormal clotting.

PATIENTS WHOSE COVID-19 was minimally symptomatic or even asymptomatic will still be vulnerable to abnormal clotting. Abnormal clotting commonly manifests as clots in the leg, clots in the lungs, or in the brain. These are known respectively as deep vein thromboses (DVT), pulmonary emboli (PE), and stroke.

THESE ARE KNOWN COLLECTIVELY as TED or thromboembolic disease. For this reason, during this COVID-19 pandemic, those who do phone triage have to be increasingly aware of reports of symptoms such as headache, pain in the calf, the leg or the medial thigh. Pain of this nature can mean that there is a clot in the veins of the leg. Clots of this nature can break off and embolize, traveling to the lungs, and this is life-threatening.

PULMONARY EMBOLI MAY PRESENT as chest pain, shortness of breath, and a feeling of dread. Thromboembolic phenomena of this nature are not that common in a young healthy population. However, *OBGYNs have to keep thromboembolic disease firmly in mind because we commonly deal with pregnant women and prescribe oral contraceptive pills, both of which add to thromboembolic risk.*

. . .

PREGNANT AND POSTPARTUM women are relatively more hypercoagulable compared to their non-pregnant counterparts. Add to this even a low-grade COVID infection, and it is not surprising that the incidence of thromboembolic disease increases in this population. The medical assistant doing phone triage bears all this in mind as she listens to patients' reports.

SOMETIMES PATIENTS who are seen regularly will call for things that are far out of the purview of an obstetrician gynecologist. Even for these things, the medical assistant needs to be alert and responsive. Women come to the OBGYN more often than they come to any other doctor, even if they have an internist, a family doctor or other subspecialists.

IT IS OFTEN the OBGYN's phone number that will first jump to mind in the wake of an emergency. Examples would include a patient calling immediately after an auto accident, a patient calling after she or another family member experiences loss of consciousness or seizure, a patient who has just experienced trauma such as falling off a horse, a patient calling after she or another member of the family has ingested something hazardous, or even a patient calling in after an assault, sexual or otherwise. (These are all actual examples from my practice.)

THE MEDICAL ASSISTANT needs to have thought through these possibilities and have quick access to her physician, but also phone numbers for Poison Control, a help crisis line, and the number to call if an ambulance needs to be dispatched.

Generally, 911 is the best option. Sometimes the patient on the other end of the line needs help remembering this. *When crisis strikes, patients and their relatives can become profoundly confused, and a quick phone call to a trusted OBGYN office is just what they need.*

COMMUNICATION AND THE MA

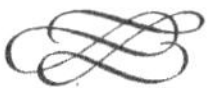

A lengthy exposition on general communications skills is outside the scope of this work. However, medical communication has certain special features. Medical communication demands a higher degree of clarity and completeness than everyday conversation. The health of the patients and the integrity of the practice depends on it.

To these ends, a few consistently used communication techniques will serve. First, it is important that the staff be good listeners. This applies to both clinical and nonclinical staff members. In particular, active listening should be the rule. Active listening entails putting your complete attention on the speaker while they are speaking. Once the message is delivered, the message is read back. In social conversation, read back might seem boorish, whereas in medical conversation, it can be life-saving. To read back is to accurately summarize what the person has just said to you. They then can confirm that they have been accurately heard.

. . .

ACTIVE LISTENING IS *a form of closed loop communication.* There are many messages going back-and-forth in a medical office. There must be confirmation that each of these reaches their destination. For example, an important result might come in and the patient must be informed of it. However, when the medical assistant called to speak with her about it, she reached only the answering machine. The MA would undoubtedly know that she should not leave sensitive medical information on the answering machine. However, the message needed delivery, so she left a message asking the patient to call the office. That would seem like enough. However, it is not. In this instance, the MA should try again the next day, and the next day again if necessary. In our office, if you try three times and do not reach the patient, a registered letter must be sent.

THIS IS COSTLY AND CUMBERSOME. That is why at the beginning of the registration for the visit, good phone numbers, alternate phone numbers, emails, and alternate persons to notify are recorded. Most of the time, a registered letter can be avoided. The communications loop must be closed, lest there be harm or liability.

A THIRD BASIC communication principle is to know your listener. In the medical clinic setting, this means, of course, being aware of their level of medical literacy. However, it also means to take non-verbal cues. Is your listener in a hurry? Are they anxious? Knowledge of these things will help you deliver your message as effectively as possible.

COMMUNICATION WITH PATIENTS

Communication between the medical assistant and the patient begins with verbal and nonverbal messages of welcome. The medical assistant becomes good at observing the patients because she sees them one after another, day in and day out. Unconsciously, she learns to stratify and categorize them in what amounts to a taxonomy of types.

From the trophy wives to the drug abusing sex workers, they all should be welcomed and put at ease. They all hold their surprises and virtues; they all have their needs with which we may be able to help. *It is at this stage that we caregivers must remember that we are privileged to have our education and to have these jobs of meaningful service.*

SIMILAR TO THE structure of the medical history, the medical assistant begins with open-ended questions and quickly focuses the conversation on the history that she must take and record. Her communication with the patient soon becomes formulaic. Despite this, the MA should remember that the patient feels like she has just made a friend, an ally. The patient will remember not just the front office person and the doctor. She will remember the medical assistant as well.

SOMETIMES MEDICAL ASSISTANTS take calls from patients which are not pertaining to medical triage. Staff must always try to "start with yes", or some supportive affirmative version of an answer. It can be challenging though, because sometimes people make unreasonable demands. For example, a patient might call in saying..." Can you work in my annual in

15 minutes?" Staff are tempted to answer with a "No, hell no." Instead, she can say something like, "We would love to help you. What is going on?" This approach is much more likely to get to the heart of the matter.

COMMUNICATION WITH DOCTORS

While the doctor and the medical assistant are, in many ways, joined at the hip, they still need to be efficient with their communication. By efficient, I mean both accurate and quick. **Medical assistants should set the pace for the doctor.** She prepares the patient in a timely fashion and notifies the doctor that the patient is ready. The MA then presents the patient to the doctor. This is a formal matter which takes a stereotypical form. We detailed this earlier, but it bears repeating. I call it "The OBGYN Preamble".

PRESENTING information to an OBGYN provider should always begin with this preamble. It includes the age, gravity, parity, and either the gestational age if pregnant, or the date of the last menstrual period if not. From there follows the chief complaint. That should be all that is necessary. The MA and the doctor may have to remind one another whether the patient needs to be undressed from the waist down, or if any consent forms or other paperwork is necessary. In this setting, reminders are always good and they can certainly be bidirectional.

COMMUNICATION WITH FELLOW MAS

Two medical assistants may be operating in tandem, so their communication during one clinic may be more administrative. However, if two medical assistants operate in series, there must be a clinical handoff. Handoff simply means the transfer of information from one medical caregiver to another, so that nothing in the patient care process is missed. For example, if one medical assistant works mornings, and her partner works afternoons, there will be some patient care activity that will span the whole day. Any concerning cases or unreturned results of concern must be discussed as the responsibilities are transferred.

SOME OFFICES MAY CHOOSE to handle this with a brief huddle, which may or may not include the doctor. *Handoff errors and omissions account for a considerable percent of medicolegal problems and patient harms.* Handoff can be verbal and written. It should not rely entirely on what is in the chart. The new MA might not look in the chart. Any concerning cases have to be called to the attention of the incoming MA. Making handoff a priority saves time and trouble.

COMMUNICATION WITH OUTSIDE OFFICES

Medical assistants have to field inquiries from other offices. Normally, this falls to the manager. Anyone who answers these calls must remember that a medical office is a business, and that helpfulness is good customer service. This includes helpfulness to another staff person in a competing office. Word gets around. *Professionalism and courtesy on the phone go a long way toward establishing a good reputation for the office in the community.*

COMMUNICATION WITH THE FRONT OFFICE

Communication between the front office and medical assistants is a two-way system. The front office, over time, has devised the schedule for the day. The medical assistant reviews it, prepares for it, and then moves the patients in and out, trying to stay on time. If something unexpected should happen in the back, such as a procedure taking longer than expected, it is the duty of the medical assistant to let the front know, so the front office person can manage expectations of the subsequent patients. Likewise, if there is a cancellation, or a need to fit someone into the schedule urgently, the front needs to let the back know as soon as possible, so the pace and possibly the room arrangement can be adjusted.

COMMUNICATIONS WITH GROUPS: MEETINGS

Group communication amounts to meetings. I am a big fan of the weekly office meeting. I am also a fan of the short structured meeting. Meetings may cover agenda items not directly related to the MA. However, each member of the office team must understand that their functioning and performance sit in the context of the whole office's performance. No matter who she is, she must understand that she is interdependent on all the other staff at the office. This is true whether the staff member is medical or administrative. While the workings of the revenue cycle do not, at first glance, seem germane to the way the front office or the medical assistants do their work, it turns out that it is. Meetings are a chance for staff members to "see how the other side lives". Meetings are a chance for one section of the office to talk to the other sections of the office about what they need to perform optimally.

MEETINGS ARE ALSO a formal early warning system on problems. It is critical that meetings constitute a safe space where challenges can be shared and problem solving can take place. Since a high functioning office has regular meetings, it provides an appropriate channel for what would otherwise be water cooler talk. Urgent matters in the office can go any time to the physician or the head MA. However, most issues can be put on the agenda for the meeting.

MEETINGS CAN BE MADE short and sweet by several procedures, and they are all derivations and simplifications of Robert's Rules. First, an agenda should be established. Anyone in the office should be able to add to it. There should, however, be a deadline for submissions to the agenda. Since meetings are weekly, the deadline can be pretty close to the meeting. Out of courtesy for the office manager, it should not be left to the day before the meeting. Therefore, agenda items should be given to the office manager two days before the meeting. The day before the meeting, the manager writes and publishes the agenda to everyone in the office. It should take the same format every time. A meeting agenda should be a sparse document on one page which shows the date and the time of the meeting, the invitees, and the format. The agenda should run something like this:

1. THE FIRST ITEM is review and approval of the last meeting minutes.

2. The second set of items are section reports, and these can be arranged any way the office sees fit. For example, there is usually a manager's report. The head MA can give an MA report. Revenue should give a report. Each report should present problems and progress.

3. The next agenda item is new business, and this comprises all the new items recently put on the agenda.

4. Actionable items are reviewed and assigned to specific people.

5. The next meeting time is established, and the meeting is adjourned.

6. The manager gets the meeting minutes out to all the invitees the next day.

THE VALUE of the meeting is in the discussion and the decision making. After each section report, or each new agenda item, a little time, for example, five minutes, of discussion can take place. If more time is needed, breakout subgroups can be created. During discussion, problems are discussed as group issues, not personal issues. Everyone is there to problem solve and make plans.

ALL THOSE ATTENDING meetings should make suggestions that conform to the SMART goals format. Smart is an acronym that stands for specific, measurable, achievable, realistic, and time bound. The suggestion "We should really be faster in clinic" is not specific, nor is it time bound. The suggestion, "By the beginning of next month, we should strive to have most of the patients for room 2 ready by the time the doctor comes out of room 1." meets these criteria. It is very specific. It is measurable. To measure it, the manager will probably have to make a spreadsheet for the MAs to fill in as they go, patient by patient, day by day. It is achievable and realistic. It also has a time goal. Interval tallies may need to be done to see if the goal is being approached. If there is inadequate progress on the goal, then a course correction can be made.

GOOD COMMUNICATION in a medical office is arguably one of the biggest determinants of patient safety and office efficiency. Quality communication must take place with staff and patients, both individually and in meetings.

AN OUNCE of prevention prevents a pound of cure. Meetings are prevention. Prevention it's not as difficult as it sounds. It is not willpower, skill, or a good memory. It is a strategy that is put into place, enacted, iterated, and refined repeatedly.

ONBOARDING

When a new employee is hired, there is a need for onboarding. Onboarding is a formal type of communication that is both verbal and written. A detailed discussion on onboarding is beyond the scope of this document. However, in a nutshell, onboarding should include three things:

1. A personal meeting with coworkers

2. A concise packet containing information on schedule and compensation, and a copy of the employment contract, which details the job description and duties.

3. Orientation to more detailed resources like lab and SOP (standard operating procedure) manuals located physically in the office and online.

. . .

THE PACKET of information should make it possible for the medical assistant to know exactly what is expected of them and when. This protects both parties. If excessive demands are made by the office, the employee can refer to the packet and her contract. If the employee is not fulfilling her responsibilities, the employer can do the same. Reviewing the contractual details should be the basis for a fruitful discussion about the way forward. Ideally, such paperwork should become a resource for success, instead of a bludgeon.

THERE IS a debate whether an employment contract is necessary for a medical assistant. I would argue that it is a good idea. An employment agreement is an opportunity to document the employee's demographics, their date of hire, and a detailed job description and terms of employment. These include not only expectations of performance but also protocols for time off, sick leave, and termination. Specifying these terms is a case of strong fences making good neighbors.

EMPLOYERS SHOULD CONSIDER a check in with the local state or county job office. I have found that these people are an underutilized and precious resource for employers, especially small ones. They have up to the minute accurate information on all the dos and don'ts of having employees. They also have printed material and online resources which will keep you and your office on the up and up.

ONBOARDING PREVENTS problems by establishing clear expectations, both administratively and professionally. It gives a new employee resources to answer her future questions which will invariably arise.

MENTORING

Mentoring is a time-honored, formal type of communication. It pairs a new with an experienced employee in the same division. Both parties must understand what mentoring is and what it is not. The relationship is not a supervisor assistant relationship. It is not primarily a relationship for evaluation. It is not competitive. It is not meant to make one employee the same as the other. Instead, the mentor is supposed to be a permissive teaching resource for the new hire. The new hires finds her own way and reaches out to the mentor as needed. The mentor may also make suggestions outright, which the new employee should strongly consider trying. In the end, however, the new hire should decide on her own way to do things as long as she fulfills her job responsibilities.

TYPICALLY, mentoring falls to the head medical assistant. Even if there are only two medical assistants, there's usually one with seniority. This leadership structure can help prevent ambiguity and establish a chain of responsibility leading, as always, to the caregiver.

MANUALS AND CHECKLISTS

Manuals need to be made and finished. However, that does not mean that they never change. All manuals in the front or the back office should take the form of a three-ring binder so that things can be added and subtracted. Similarly, the content in all manuals needs to be created and kept in a digital form for two reasons. First, this enables it to be easily edited. Second, it can be uploaded to a common site such as a Google Drive for everyone to access it anywhere and anytime.

REQUISITE MANUALS in a medical office include but are not limited to: the front office manual, the medical assistant manual, the laboratory manual, and the revenue cycle manual. The respective staff in each office section should make their own manual. All the manuals should be edited for accuracy by the manager and the physician. All editions should be dated and initialed.

MANUALS MUST CONTAIN CHECKLISTS. For example, the medical assistant's manual will contain a page about setting up for and assisting with a colposcopy. The list of supplies for the procedure should be in a small laminated checklist that can be removed and taken into the room. This is far less bulky and obtrusive than bringing the whole manual into the room. Those responsible for making their section's manual should always be on the lookout for what can be made into a list. List making is now recognized as an art unto itself and can greatly enhance performance.

CHECKLISTS MAY BE BROUGHT out for procedures, but they should be stored out of the patient's view. The patient does not need to sit alone in a room on an exam table and contemplate a card on the wall which lists betadine, anesthetic spray, scalpel or small sharp scissors, pickups with teeth, and silver nitrate cautery sticks. By the same logic, the patient does not need to gaze over the receptionist's shoulder to see a sticky note saying, "It is imperative that you ask the patient to pay any past balances, to pay her co-pay, and to make payments on her anticipated deductible. Remind her that we take cash, local checks, and all credit cards."

MANUALS, checklists, and posterized reminders or sticky notes belong in a medical office. The patient, however, should not be subjected to them. Her experience should be tranquil and spa-like as much as possible.

PERFORMANCE REVIEWS AND PROBATION

All staff should have regular performance reviews. Performance reviews give staff feedback and opportunity to improve. They also give leadership an opportunity to give props those staff doing a good job. The knowledge that performance reviews are done will help keep some staff on their toes. Performance reviews inform benefits. Performance reviews should always be done in a spirit of empowering the employee to become better. The blame and shame approach has long been discredited as ineffective.

IDENTIFYING problems with MAs is not as easy as it sounds. Rarely is someone materially deficient in their performance, i.e., bad with procedures, rude to patients, or completely incapable of charting. Medical Assistants as a group are mission driven professionals who choose their position mindfully. However, they, like the rest of us, are not immune to the vicissitudes of life and can get dragged down, sometimes without even realizing it themselves. This sort of thing can even happen outside of the view of the physician since the MA may feel her best when she is working directly alongside the physician.

A STRUGGLING medical assistant may manifest in any of the following ways: a general feeling of stress or unhappiness around the office, increased patient complaints or departures, or even charting and resultant billing issues that grow out of her work.

OCCASIONALLY, a staff person needs to be put on probation for significant and repeated problems not responsive to feedback. A probationary meeting should be scheduled with two staff members and the employee. At the time of the probationary meeting, the staff person needs to be given terms of the probation, including the list of concerns, their solutions, and a time frame to meet each one. She deserves as much specificity as possible, in a full SMART goal format. She should also, within reason, be given the resources she needs to be successful.

CONCLUSION: RELATIONSHIPS MAKE THE OFFICE

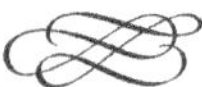

What makes for a great medical office? Is it science? Educated staff? Is it lots of money, technology and great architecture? Is it friendly people? Of course it is all these things and more. If you take science, education, money, technology, architecture, and people, you don't have a great medical office until you add healthy work relationships. Healthy work relationships are the foundation of good patient care and a great work environment. This is because great patient care and a pleasant work environment depend on accurate and effective communication.

ONE OF THE most advanced forms of communication is civil disagreement. That is, disagreement which is clear, constructive and even collaborative. Staff members in the medical clinic need to have the freedom and safety to disagree, then troubleshoot as a group.

. . .

Great medical care is a team sport. All the players on the team are crucial and they must work together the right way. The playbook is clear. Open expression, active listening, and closed loop communication are key. Groups who are not working well should seek outside coaching as the need arises.

A lot about medicine is algorithmic. A lot about being a medical assistant is algorithmic. Checklists and reminders are germane to most of what the medical assistant does. However, medical care is also full of surprises. Any patient, however seemingly normal, can throw a serious curveball into the clinic day. The entire staff needs to be ready to flex to meet the need. Therefore, a great clinic environment must have a healthy balance between regimentation and flexibility. Staff in both the front office and the back office must remember that they are all working toward shared goals: good patient care and a great working environment.

The medical office system has, by design, multiple moving parts. It is something that will never work perfectly. That is something that everyone should accept. If one part of the office is struggling, management and leadership should reach out in supportive curiosity to learn about the situation and see how they can help.

Once leadership and management, together with the other stakeholders, have understood the situation and made a plan, the whole office should help with course correction. And, in a form of higher level closed loop communication, the effects of the plan should be monitored and reported on at each office meeting, allowing for ongoing iterative course correction.

THE MEDICAL ASSISTANT is often at the center of this process to define challenges, devise plans, and monitor results. She is the center of the office in that she brings together the front and back offices, as well as bringing together the patient and the physician. She is the guardian of the closed loop.

A HIGH-PERFORMING medical office should incorporate the reminders in this book every day. Communication skills and a shared sense of purpose are easily forgotten during the chaos and pressure of certain clinic days. Hopefully, the insights and recommendations in this work will allow offices to function smoothly so that great care can be delivered, and so that staff can feel satisfied and supported while delivering it.

ACRONYMS IN OB/GYN

A

AAP -American Association of Pediatrics

ABOG-American Board of Obstetrics and Gynecology

ACA-Affordable Care Act

ACOG-American College of Obstetricians and Gynecologists

AMA-American Medical Association

AROM-Artificial rupture of membranes

B

BMI-Body mass index

BMP-Basic metabolic profile

C

CAT-Computed axial tomography

CBC-Complete blood count

CEO-Chief executive officer

CIN-Cervical intraepithelial neoplasia

CMP-Comprehensive metabolic profile

CNA-Certified nursing assistant

COLPO-Colposcopy

CT-Chlamydia trachomatis

CX-Cervix

D

DDX-Differential diagnosis

DVT-Deep vein thrombosis

E

EBV-Epstein Barr virus

EFM-External fetal monitor

EMB-Endometrial biopsy

EMR-Electronic medical record

F

FLU-Influenza

G

GBS-Group B strep

GC-Gonococcus

GI-Gastrointestinal

GU-Genitourinary

H

HBV-Hepatitis B virus

HCG-Human chorionic gonadotropin

HCV-Hepatitis C virus

HDL-High density lipoprotein

HELLP-Hemolysis, elevation of liver functions, and low platelets

HIPAA-Health insurance, portability, and accountability act

HIV-Human immunodeficiency virus

HPI-History of present illness

HPV-Human papillomavirus

HSV1- Herpes simplex virus type one

HSV2- Herpes simplex virus type two

I

IDK- I don't know

IUD- Intrauterine device

L

LDL- Low density lipoprotein

LEEP- Loop electrical excision procedure

LPN- Licensed professional nurse

M

MA- Medical assistant

MRI - Magnetic resonance imaging

MULTIP- Multiparous patient

N

NIPS- Non invasive prenatal screening

NST- Non stress test

O

OP - Occiput posterior

OSA- Obstructive sleep apnea

P

PAP- Papanicolaou smear

PCOS- Polycystic ovarian syndrome

PCR- Polymerase chain reaction

PE- PE can refer to both physical exam and pulmonary embolism

PMH- Past medical history

PPROM- Preterm premature rupture of membranes

PRIMIP- Primiparous patient

PSH- Past surgical history

R

RBCA- Risks, benefits, complications, and alternatives

RH- Rhesus

RHOGAM- Rho(D) immune globulin (human)

RN-Registered nurse

ROM-Rupture of membranes

ROS- Review of systems

RPR-Rapid plasma reagin, a test for syphilis

RSV-Respiratory syncytial virus

S

SMART-Specific, measurable, attainable, relevant, and time bound

SOAP-Subjective, objective, assessment and plan (a note format)

STS-Serologic tests for syphilis

T

TDAP- Tetanus, diphtheria, and a cellular pertussis

TED- Thromboembolic disease

TOA-Tubo ovarian abscess

TOCO-Tocodynamometer, a device that indirectly measures the strength of the uterine contractions from the surface of the abdomen

TOXO-Toxoplasmosis

U

UC-Uterine contractions

URI-Upper respiratory infection

UTI-Urinary tract infection

V

VAIN-Vaginal intraepithelial neoplasia

VIN-Vulvar intraepithelial neoplasia

VOC-Volatile organic compounds

VS-Vital signs

VSS-Vital signs stable

VZV-Varicella zoster virus

W

WADAO-Weak and dizzy, all over

WNL-Within normal limits

GLOSSARY

A

Abscess: an infected collection of pus

Adnexal: Pertaining to the adnexa, which are the pelvic organs to each side of the uterus, the tubes, ovaries and the tissue and ligaments planes connecting them.

Affordable Care Act (ACA): A comprehensive health care reform law enacted in March 2010, aimed at expanding health insurance coverage, controlling health care costs, and improving the health care delivery system in the United States. It aimed to insure people who did not qualify for Medicaid, but who could not afford private insurance.

Abnormal uterine bleeding (AUB): A condition involving irregular, excessive, or unpredictable menstrual bleeding, which requires an evaluation, particularly in patients with specific risk factors or during menopause.

Algorithm: a pattern, plan, or protocol for accomplishing something. Adjective form is algorithmic. The opposite approach would be to decide in the moment.

American College of Obstetricians and Gynecologists (ACOG): A leading organization in the field of obstetrics and gynecology, providing guidelines and recommendations for screening and procedures, including those related to social history inquiries.

Amniocentesis: the retrieval of fluid via the ultrasound, guided insertion of a needle. This is commonly used to obtain genetic material of the baby. Noninvasive prenatal testing (NIPS) has made this procedure rarer.

Anaphylaxis: a life-threatening allergic reaction which can lead to respiratory and circulatory collapse

Anxiety: A common patient reaction to medical procedures, often stemming from concerns about discomfort, costs, and potential diagnoses; caregivers and medical assistants play a key role in mitigating this through preparation, communication, and support.

Anxiolytic: Medication to treat anxiety

Appy: Colloquial term for appendectomy, a surgical procedure to remove the appendix, with specific notation required in the patient's chart if the appendix was ruptured at the time of operation due to implications for future surgeries.

Atrial Fibrillation (Afib): An irregular and often abnormally rapid heartbeat generated in the atria or top chambers of the heart.

B

Betadine: A common antiseptic used in medical procedures for which patients should be screened for allergies to avoid adverse reactions. Patients allergic to shellfish should be suspected of iodine and Betadine allergy.

Bigeminy: A heart rhythm where two beats occur very close to one another. Does consist of a PVC alternating with a single sinus beat.

Body Mass Index (BMI): A measure used to determine obesity or underweight by calculating a ratio of height to weight, with specific implications for patient care and monitoring in medical practices.

Biopsy: The removal of a small piece of tissue for examination under a microscope to check for disease.

Blood type: Blood type refers to the main antigen identification system of the red blood cells. Antigens are surface features of the red blood cells. The most important antigens on the human red blood cells are the ABO antigens. In adult humans there are types A, B, O, and AB. There are other antigen systems on the surface of human red blood cells. The second most well-known is the Rh system where the cells can either be Rh positive or Rh negative.

Boutique Style Practice: A medical practice offering personalized and continuous care, often with a focus on patient experience and higher autonomy for staff.

Bradycardia: a low heart rate, typically under 60 bpm for an adult.

C

Certified Nursing Assistant (CNA): A certified professional who provides basic care to patients, assisting them with daily activities under the supervision of a registered nurse (RN) or licensed practical nurse (LPN).

Cervical Dysplasia: Abnormal growth of cells on the surface of the cervix, often detected through Pap smears and potentially requiring procedures like colposcopy for further evaluation.

Cervix: The end of the uterus facing the vagina. It is histologically distinct from the uterus and is therefore subject to different disease processes.

Chaperone: an attendant of various types who witnesses and documents the communications and procedures in a room between a healthcare provider and a patient

Chief Complaint (CC): The primary issue or symptom reported by a patient during a medical visit, serving as a crucial element in guiding the direction of clinical assessment and care.

Chlamydia: A common sexually transmitted organism. Testing is recommended for women, particularly in their twenties, to detect chlamydia infection, which can cause pelvic infection, pain, fallopian tube scarring, and infertility. It can cause serious potential complications in pregnancy and for newborns.

Colposcopy: A diagnostic procedure involving the examination of the cervix, vagina or perineum with a colposcope. It is done following certain abnormal Pap smear results to identify areas of abnormality for biopsy.

Condyloma: see genital warts

Consent: The process of informing a patient about the risks, benefits, complications, and alternatives of a procedure, ensuring their understanding and agreement before proceeding.

Constipation: uncomfortable, or infrequent, bowel movements. A person is considered constipated when bowel movements result in passage of a small amount of hard, dry stool, usually fewer than three times a week.

Contraception: birth control

Cytology: The study of human cells

D

Didelphic: this pertains to uterine didelphys, which means a double uterus caused by an error in embryological development. Each side of the double uterus is smaller than normal. The cervix of such a uterus is more likely to be incompetent.

Differential Diagnosis: The list of potential conditions under consideration when a certain diagnosis is being sought.

Dysmenorrhea: pain with menstruation

Dyspareunia: pain with intercourse

Dysplasia: Abnormal cell changes in tissue that may be mild, moderate, or severe and can progress toward pre-cancer.

Dysuria: pain with urination

E

Ectocervical: Pertaining to the surface of the cervix.

Ectopic Pregnancy: A potentially life-threatening condition where a pregnancy develops unsustainably outside the uterus, often in the fallopian tubes.

Eclampsia: a variant of severe preeclampsia which includes seizures

Electronic Medical Record (EMR): A digital version of a patient's paper chart that contains the medical and treatment history

Endemic: regularly occurring within a restricted community

Endocervical: Pertaining to the cervical canal

Endometrial Biopsy (EMB): An office procedure in which a small sample of the lining of the uterus (endometrium) is collected for microscopic examination, typically to investigate abnormal uterine bleeding.

Electrolytes: the inorganic ions in the serum, such as sodium, potassium, and chloride

Electronic Medical Record (EMR): A digital version of a patient's medical history, improving the efficiency of data storage, retrieval, and sharing across healthcare providers.

Epidemic: rapid spread of a condition in a restricted community

Evidence-based: this is a description of a concept, practice, or procedure based on verifiable scientific evidence rather than subjective experience.

Expectation setting: Expectation setting is the process of establishing clear and realistic expectations among individuals about what can be achieved, delivered, or expected in a given situation. It involves communicating goals, timelines, roles, and responsibilities to ensure everyone is on the same page and working towards a common objective.

F

Fallopian Tubes: Tubes coming from the upper end of the uterus through which an egg travels from the ovary to the interior of the uterus

False negative: a test which comes back negative, but in truth, is positive.

False positive: a test which comes back positive, but in truth, is not.

Family History (FH): A record of medical information about a patient's relatives, providing insights into potential hereditary conditions or predispositions.

Fibroids: also known as myomas, which are smooth, benign muscle growths of the uterus.

Follicle: When pertaining to women's health, usually refers to the immature egg stored in the ovary.

Follicular phase: the time of the menstrual cycle between day one and ovulation. It is so named because it is the time during which the follicle is maturing. Its length can can vary widely, but is usually about 14 days.

Formalin: this is a clear liquid tissue preservative, commonly used to transport biopsies to the laboratory.

G

Genital warts: Also known as condyloma, they are a manifestation of human papilloma virus. They are sexually transmitted. They can be treated with a variety of ablative and excision techniques.

Gestational diabetes: the development of diabetes in pregnancy, with consequences to both mother and baby

Glucola testing: this is a 50 g load of sugar given to patients to test for gestational diabetes at 28 weeks, also called a one hour glucola.

Glucose tolerance test: this is a three hour test involving a fasting blood sugar, a 100 g glucose load, followed by a 1 hour, a two hour and a three hour test of blood sugar. Exceeding the limits on two of the four tests constitutes a fail, and confirms a diagnosis of gestational diabetes.

Gonorrhea: This is a sexually transmitted infection which can cause serious illness in the pelvis and beyond. It also has serious implications for pregnancy.

Gravida: literally a pregnant woman, but often used to show the number of times a woman has been pregnant

Group B strep (GBS): this is a common bacterium carried as flora in the reproductive tracts of approximately 20% of women. It can cause serious disease in the newborn and the postpartum woman. Screening is routinely performed for Group B strep at 35 weeks of gestation.

H

hCG (human chorionic gonadotropin): the so-called pregnancy hormone is an easily measured artifact of pregnancy which rises predictably during early pregnancy. Pregnancies which seem unstable can be tracked by serial measurements of hCG.

HELLP syndrome: this is a severe variant of preeclampsia, comprising hemolysis, elevation of liver function tests, and low platelets. Seizure prophylaxis with magnesium and immediate delivery are indicated.

Hibiclens: a commonly used surgical cleanser, which is an alternative to iodine-based Betadine, for those who have iodine allergies.

Histology: The study of human tissues.

HIV (human immunodeficiency virus): this is a virus that causes AIDS.

Hyperemesis Gravidarium: Severe nausea and vomiting in pregnancy that can lead to dehydration and require hospitalization.

Hospital Consolidation: The process by which smaller hospitals are acquired by larger health systems or merge with other hospitals, often leading to fewer independent practitioners.

Human Papilloma virus (HPV): A common sexually transmitted virus with multiple subtypes, some of which can cause genital warts and cervical cancer.

Hypertension: High blood pressure

Hypoxia: low blood oxygen typically less than 94% on room air

I

Incompetent cervix: a cervix, which is abnormal in form, and or function, predisposing a patient to miscarriage, second semester loss, or preterm labor. An incompetent cervix can be present from birth or after surgery on the cervix. It can also be caused by damage during a vaginal delivery.

Intrauterine Device (IUD): A small, often T-shaped birth control device inserted into the uterus during an office procedure. IUDs can be hormonal or non-hormonal.

K

Kidney function tests: There are many, but commonly performed office tests include BUN and creatinine, which are available on a basic metabolic profile.

L

Labia: These are the flap like structures on either side of the vaginal opening, which protect it from the external environment. Closest to the vaginal opening are the thin labia minora. More lateral toward the leg are the larger labia majora.

Lichen sclerosis: an important and relatively common vulvar disease, characteristically presenting with itchy, dry patches, and agglutination of the vulvar structures. Diagnosis requires biopsy.

Lidocaine: a common local anesthetic used as a cream or an injectable

Lipids: the collection of fats circulating in serum, including the various types of cholesterol such as HDL and LDL, as well as triglycerides.

Lugol's solution: This is an iodine based solution used during colposcopy, to more easily visualize abnormal tissue on the surface of the cervix. Lugol's solution can stain normal tissue brown, but dysplastic tissue remains nonstaining, and appears light colored compared to the Lugols stained normal tissue. Applying Lugol's solution to the cervix makes abnormal tissue stand out. This can help guide the location of biopsies taken at the time of colposcopy.

Luteal phase: the time of the menstrual cycle between ovulation and the first day of the next menstrual period. It is so named because the corpus luteum is actively producing progesterone. The length of the luteal phase is always 14 days.

M

Medical Assistant (MA): A licensed health care professional who supports the work of physicians and other health professionals, usually in a clinic setting.

Menorrhagia: Excessively heavy or prolonged menstrual bleeding

Menometrorrhagia: Periods which are abnormal in both flow and timing.

Mise en Place: A concept borrowed from French cooking, meaning to put in place. It refers to the preparation and organization required before performing medical procedures, ensuring efficiency and reducing the risk of errors.

Mononucleosis: A febrile illness common and typically mild in young children, but more significant in an older population. It is caused by Epstein-Barr virus. As with other viruses of its class, the herpesvirus family, it may have lingering complications.

Mullerian abnormalities: abnormalities of the female reproductive tract generated during embryonic growth. Primitive reproductive structures in the female are called mullerian. Examples are heart shaped uterus, and uterine didelphys.

Myalgias: muscle aches. These are typically seen with influenza A or B, Covid, or flare of autoimmunity.

Noninvasive prenatal testing (NIPS): this is the screening of pregnant women using a blood draw, which can identify fetal cells and evaluate them for genetic and other abnormalities.

Neural tube defects: These comprise a spectrum of abnormalities where the neural tube, which surrounds the spinal cord, does not completely close during development. Neural tube defects can be prevented by adequate folic acid in early pregnancy. Prenatal vitamins are specially formulated to address this concern.

O

Obesity: a body mass index over 30

Obstetrician Gynecologist (OBGYN): A physician and surgeon specializing in women's reproductive health, including pregnancy, childbirth, and disorders of the reproductive system.

Onboarding: The process of installing a new employee into a new workplace. It involves introducing them to coworkers, educating them as to their responsibilities, assigning mentors and supervisors and providing access to manuals and operational systems.

Orthostatic vital signs: vital signs taken supine (laying down), sitting up, and standing. Both pulse and blood pressure must be taken in all three positions.

Osteopenia: low bone density, with a T score between -1.5 and -2.5.

Osteoporosis: very low bone density, with a T score less than -2.5.

P

Pandemic: Rapid spread of a condition over a country or beyond

Pap Smear: A screening procedure for cervical cancer in which cells from the cervix are collected and sent for examination.

Para: the number of times someone has given birth

Past Medical History (PMH): A comprehensive record of a patient's health issues, treatments, and outcomes, essential for informed clinical decision-making.

Pelvic inflammatory disease (PID): This common misnomer refers to an infection in the pelvis, including any or all of the pelvic organs. It is more extensive than a cervicitis, which is restricted to the cervix, and can make a patient seriously ill, including causing sepsis.

Pertinent negatives: Elements of the medical history which, by their confirmed absence, help determine the diagnosis. For example, the absence of pain helps rule out appendicitis. Here, the absence of pain is a pertinent negative.

Pertinent positives: elements of the medical history, which, by their confirmed presence, help determine the diagnosis. For example, the presence of fever helps confirm the diagnosis of appendicitis. In this case, presence of fever is a pertinent positive.

Phlebotomy: the drawing of blood.

Pick ups: these are tweezer like surgical instruments of various weights and lengths, with, and without teeth, which are small protrusions at the end meant to aid in holding onto slippery tissues.

Pipelle: This is a slim plastic straw like device with a plunger on the inside. It typically has measurement hash marks and is used to insert inside the uterus to retrieve a specimen of endometrium.

Polymerase Chain Reaction (PCR) Assay: A sensitive laboratory technique used to detect specific DNA sequences, such as those of HPV, aiding in the diagnosis and management of related conditions.

Preeclampsia: A part of the spectrum of hypertensive disorders of pregnancy, it is an inflammatory and immune mediated disorder involving high blood pressure, swelling, and disturbances to various organ systems, especially the kidney, brain and placenta. It is an indication for immediate evaluation and often delivery. Severe forms involve disturbances of liver function and clotting. This is called HELLP syndrome (see HELLP). When seizure occurs as a part of preeclampsia, it is called eclampsia.

Preterm Labor: Labor that begins before 37 weeks of pregnancy, potentially resulting in premature birth.

Private Practice OBGYN: An OBGYN who operates independently, owning their practice rather than being employed by a hospital or health system.

Procedure: A medical or surgical intervention performed for diagnostic or therapeutic purposes, requiring informed consent and careful preparation by the healthcare team.

Q

Q10 effect: This is the measured effect of an increase in temperature of 10°F on metabolism, most commonly pulse.

R

Residency: The period of a doctor's training after medical school and the receipt of the medical doctor degree. It pertains to their specialization and is typically between three and seven years long.

Rh status: This refers to the antigen system of the human red blood cells wherein cells can either be Rh positive or Rh negative. 85% of people are Rh positive. Women who are Rh negative may carry Rh positive babies. This may provoke an immune attack on the red blood cells of the baby. However, this can be prevented by a shot of Rh immunoglobulin during the pregnancy. The shot is called Rhogam.

RhoGAM: A shot given to pregnant women with Rh-negative blood to prevent Rh incompatibility issues with a fetus or newborn.

Risk Factors: Conditions or behaviors that increase the likelihood of developing a disease or adverse health outcome, critical for patient assessment and management.

Robert's Rules: A formal published protocol for the conduct of a meeting **Round ligaments:** These are ligaments coming from the top corners of the front of the uterus and inserting in the right and left groins. They are prone to painful stretching in the second trimester of pregnancy.

S

Screening test: This is a test designed to be the first step in an evaluation. The ability to sensitively detect a condition is the most important characteristic of a screening test. This sensitivity may be at the expense of specificity. This means that a screening test may have a tendency to over diagnose a condition. Later testing can determine whether the initial screening test result was true or false. The second important characteristic of a screening test is low cost, conferring a low barrier to utilization.

Scribing: The process by which a healthcare professional, such as a medical assistant, documents the physician's encounter with patients in real-time, allowing doctors to focus on patient care.

Sensitivity and Specificity: Metrics used to evaluate the accuracy of diagnostic tests, with sensitivity measuring the test's ability to correctly identify those with the disease and specificity measuring the ability to exclude those without the disease.

Sepsis: a life-threatening systemic infection which has entered the bloodstream and threatens cardiovascular integrity and major organ systems.

Sleep hygiene: Broadly speaking, this involves the practices employed to optimize sleep. These include behavior during the day, which will influence sleep in the night, such as caffeine consumption, alcohol consumption, timing of meals and exercise, as well as sleep and wake times.

SMART goals: An acronym for an effective protocol for achieving goals. See Acronym List.

Social History (SH): An assessment of a patient's lifestyle, habits, and social environment, providing context for health risks, and informing tailored care strategies.

Sphygmomanometer: A blood pressure cuff

Sponge on a stick: This is a ring forceps holding a tightly folded 4 x 4 gauze sponge

Steri-Strips: These are the brand name of a small, sterile bandage used to aid in wound closure

Symptom: Something a patient feels. Contrast with a sign, which is something a patient observes, such as a rash.

Syphilis: This is a serious sexually transmitted disease, which has different phases of manifestation over a period of years. It has serious consequences for mother and baby. Early detection and treatment are essential.

T

Tachycardia: A high heart rate, typically over 100 bpm for an adult.

Teratogen: A substance or infection capable of causing abnormal development in a fetus.

Tischler biopsy forceps: This is a specialized, long handled, biopsy, forceps suitable for biopsy of the cervix.

Toxoplasmosis: a parasitic infection commonly acquired from domestic cat feces. It is a known teratogen to early pregnancy. It is the reason that litter boxes should be avoided by those who are pregnant.

Transaminases: These are the commonly ordered liver function tests, such as AST and ALT, which are liver enzymes

Transparency: Transparency refers to the quality of being open, honest, and clear in all interactions, communications, and transactions. It involves sharing information, intentions, and actions in a straightforward and easily accessible manner, allowing others to understand the what, why, and how of a situation or decision.

Trigeminy: This consists of three heart beats very close together. In particular, a PVC (premature ventricular contraction) occurs after two sinus beats.

Trimester: A somewhat arbitrary division of pregnancy into three parts

U

Uterine sound: this is a straight, long, narrow, slightly blunt tipped instrument for measuring the depth of the uterine cavity. They are typically malleable, and can be slightly curved by the operator doing the procedure.

V

Vasovagal Reaction: A common physiological response to stress or certain stimuli, resulting in fainting or lightheadedness, which healthcare providers must anticipate and manage during procedures. A sudden drop in heart rate and blood pressure leading to fainting, often in response to a stressor.

Vertex: Head down position of the baby

Vulva: The region of the female perineum in between the top of the labia and the anus, comprising all the lateral tissues. Significantly, the vulva is vulnerable to the human papillomavirus, similar to the cervix. Dysplasia in this region is called those are intraepithelial neoplasia or VIN.

ABOUT THE AUTHOR

Gina Nelson is a board-certified obstetrician gynecologist and Fellow of the American College of Obstetricians and Gynecologists. She has been in continuous solo practice since 1994, when she finished residency at the University of Colorado Health Sciences Center, now known as University of Colorado Anschutz Medical Campus.

Before that, she grew up in Los Angeles, attended Stanford University, and graduated from the University of Utah School of Medicine in 1989.

Her professional interests lie in holistic OBGYN care, with an emphasis on nutrition, fitness, and general self care. She is also particularly interested in long term continuity of care in a boutique practice environment.

Dr. Nelson is fortunate to have delivered the babies of many women she delivered long ago. She calls these her professional grandchildren. At present, two of of them work alongside her in the clinic as staff.

Other professional interests have been robotic surgery and amniotic fluid embolism (AFE). In 2014, she gave a TEDx talk on AFE titled, "The Girl Who Lived".

She lives on a farm by a river with her husband of 40 years. They have three adult children and two granddaughters.

Dr. Nelson has been a lupus patient since 1994.

Her personal interests include longevity and health tracking. She enjoys a variety of sports, especially dance and TaeKwondo. She enjoys gardening and entertaining. She is a foodie and a fan of Kpop.

She can be reached at

www.drginanelson.com

Phone 406-755-6550

info@drginanelson.com

Office located in Kalispell, Montana, USA

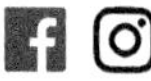